#dinewithdignity

Unlocking the Mystery of Dementia & Dining

TONI FISK

First published by Ultimate World Publishing 2021

ISBN

Paperback: 978-1-922597-21-2
Ebook: 978-1-922597-22-9

Cover design: Ultimate World Publishing
Layout and typesetting: Ultimate World Publishing
Editor: Rebecca Low
Cover photo: posteriori-Shutterstock.com

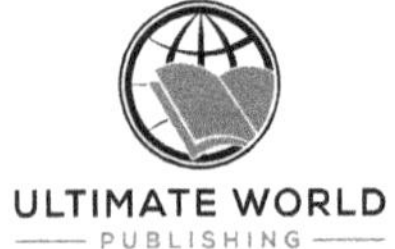

Ultimate World Publishing
Diamond Creek,
Victoria Australia 3089
www.writeabook.com.au

Testimonials

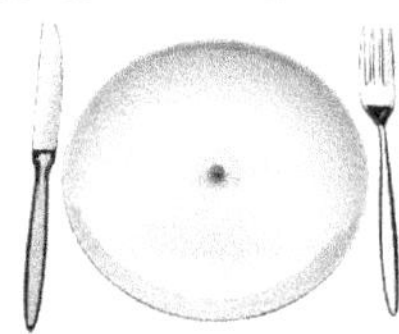

"Toni has the ability to break down complex dining models and processes into their basic elements to improve both outcomes and efficiencies. Toni's teaching and mentoring abilities enable her to unlock hidden potential from her readers."

C. Lukas,
Vice President Partnerships at HomeKook'd Inc.

"I have worked with Toni at multiple senior communities. She effortlessly provided basic dementia education and techniques to the staff members we were working with. Everyone was amazed and couldn't believe the results. Total "aha" moments. She knows her stuff, and presents with a style that is engaging, funny, and passionate. I learned so much about how to best manage not only my multiple clients' journeys with dementia, but my mother's journey as well."

M. Perisi,
Director of Dining Services Senior Living.

"I struggled with how to best understand and care for my parents, who both had dementia in their last years. This book would have been a tremendous help. I wish it had been available to guide me during that difficult time."

M. Taubenheim

"The presenter was very thorough, she covered everything I wanted to hear on dementia."

"I thank God for Mrs. Toni. Her presentation on dementia was good and clear because I was able to follow the activities that she offered."

"We really appreciate the workshop. We thank you from the bottom of our hearts."

East Meadow UMC senior Workshop

Dedication

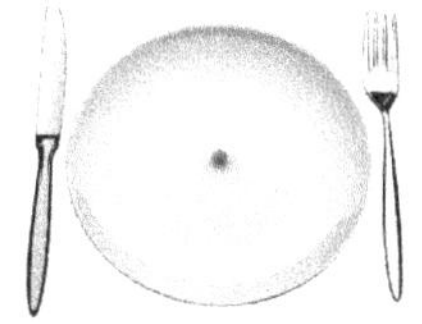

I dedicate this book to my Mom, whom I think of every day and know she is watching over me. I want to thank both my husband, Clyde Reece, and my son, Andre Reece, who willingly and consistently supported this endeavor and my dream.

Contents

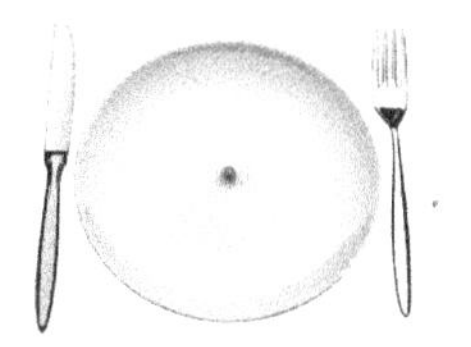

Foreword

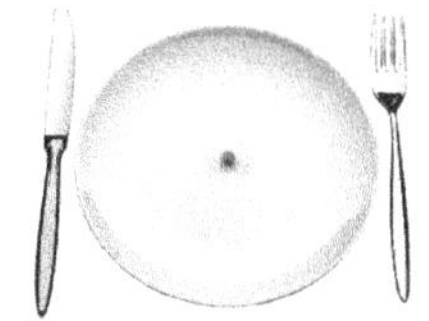

I wrote this book because it needed to be written. Currently, any fundamental and supportive information relating to dementia and dining is fragmented, lacking in detail, and scattered across the web. As a long-serving provider of Senior Living and Memory Care Dining, I was able to button up the basic, yet key components needed to assist you, the care partners of people living with dementia.

My mission was to provide the backdrop to the "why" and then delve into the "how." I did not get technical with my information as I wanted everyone to understand in clear and simple terms what you are dealing with (or about to) when caring for your loved one. At the end of the book, I will offer opportunities for you to take advantage of to further your skills and education.

I'd like to thank my Senior Living peers and other industry experts for their input in developing this book in addition to my own extensive research of evidence-based methods of engagement, documented best practices, and authentic personal experience.

As you read the book, I recommend you follow the flow of the chapters as each chapter is crammed with real-life fundamentals and appealing suggestions. One section may shout out at you to jump on first, but please be sure to read the entire book to appreciate the whole educational experience of caring for a person living with dementia.

I have taken steps to implement the teachings and trainings about dementia of Teepa Snow and the Positive Approach to Care®. I serve as a PAC™ Certified Independent Trainer Professional to guide learning and skills as supported by certification types. While inspired by my certification, all knowledge and skills offered here are only representative of me, independent of the Positive Approach to Care organization. Educational content provided by Positive Approach® is used with permission and based on the GEMS® Model and the techniques, strategies, and overall approach to care created and developed by Positive Approach, LLC. www.teepasnow.com

Medical disclaimer: Readers, please note that the content in this book and on my website is for informational or educational purposes only. It does not substitute professional medical advice or consultations with healthcare professionals as to the exact and specific care for your loved one, or persons in your care.

Chapter 1

What's Wrong With Mom?

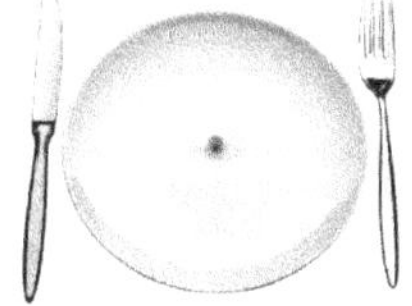

Geez Louise, what's going on with Mom? To misplace her keys (again) is one thing, but when she stands there and looks at them and cannot remember what she's supposed to do with them... well, this is a sure signal to see a neurologist—not just a general practitioner.

DON'T PANIC! Please note that sometimes lapses in memory or odd physical actions can also be driven by common medical issues. Your loved one could be experiencing the side effects of thyroid, kidney, liver, heart or lung problems, or urinary or chest infections which are among the many medical conditions that can produce dementia-like symptoms and can be corrected by proper medical attention. Sometimes people have a hard time expressing themselves, so keep an eye out for changes in routines, behavior (weepy/angry) and amounts of liquids or food being consumed.

Many of the early warning signs of dementia are also common symptoms of aging. To the untrained eye, it may seem like a combination of "senior moments." However, when several symptoms or indicators are combined with rapid onset or increasing intensity, your loved one should be screened by their physician for basic health imbalances or screened for dementia by a neurologist as soon as possible. Put on your detective hat, invest the time to discover the root cause of their actions and behaviors and do your best to not leap to the worst conclusion.

What exactly is dementia...isn't it the same as Alzheimer's disease? Dementia is a syndrome in which there is deterioration in memory, thinking, behavior and the ability to perform everyday activities. Although dementia mainly affects older people, it is not a normal part of aging.

Dementia is an umbrella term that Alzheimer's disease can fall under and can occur due to a variety of conditions. It is considered the most common form of dementia, accounting for, according to the Alzheimer's Association, 60 to 80 percent of all cases of dementia.

As dementia progresses, it can have a huge impact on the ability to function independently. It is a major cause of disability for older adults and places an emotional and financial burden on families and care partners.

The World Health Organization says that an estimated 50 million people around the world are living with dementia. These numbers are projected to reach 82 million by the year 2030 and 152 million by 2050, with the majority of individuals coming from low- and middle-income countries. Per the Alzheimer's Association, within the United States, approximately 5.7 million people are living with dementia.

You are more likely to develop dementia as you age when certain brain cells are damaged. Many conditions can cause dementia, including degenerative diseases such as Alzheimer's, Parkinson's, and Huntington's. Each cause of dementia creates damage to a different set of brain cells. The exact cause is unknown, and no cure is available.

Dementia 101 – Different Types of Dementia and Their Effects

Dementia is a term used to describe severe changes in the brain. These changes make it difficult for people to perform basic daily activities. In most people, dementia causes changes in behavior and personality. There are, under the dementia umbrella, over 100 types of dementia.

Dementia affects three areas of the brain:

- language
- memory
- decision-making

Most cases of dementia are caused by a disease and cannot be reversed. Alcohol and drug abuse can sometimes cause dementia as well. In those cases, it can be possible to reverse the damage in the brain. But, according to the Cleveland Clinic, reversal happens in fewer than 20 percent of people with dementia.

10 Types of Dementia

Alzheimer's Disease

Alzheimer's disease is the most common type of dementia. Between 60 to 80 percent of cases of dementia are caused by this disease, according to the Alzheimer's Association. Early signs of Alzheimer's disease include depression, forgetting names and recent events, and a depressed mood. However, depression is not part of Alzheimer's disease. It's a separate disorder that must be treated specifically. Occasionally, depressed older adults are misdiagnosed as having Alzheimer's disease.

Alzheimer's disease is characterized by brain cell death. As the disease progresses, people experience confusion and mood changes. They also have trouble speaking and walking.

Older adults are more likely to develop Alzheimer's. About 5 percent of cases of Alzheimer's are early-onset Alzheimer's, occurring in people in their 40s or 50s.

Vascular Dementia

The second most common type of dementia is vascular dementia. It's caused by a lack of blood flow to the brain. Vascular dementia can happen as you age and can be related to atherosclerotic disease or stroke.

Symptoms of vascular dementia can appear slowly or suddenly, depending on what's causing it. Confusion and disorientation are common early signs. Later on, people also have trouble completing tasks or concentrating for long periods of time.

Vascular dementia can cause vision problems and sometimes hallucinations as well.

Dementia with Lewy Bodies

Dementia with Lewy bodies, also known as Lewy body dementia, is caused by protein deposits in nerve cells. This interrupts chemical messages in the brain and causes memory loss and disorientation.

People with this type of dementia also experience visual hallucinations and have trouble falling asleep at night or fall asleep unexpectedly during the day. They also might faint or become lost or disoriented.

Dementia with Lewy bodies shares many symptoms with Parkinson's and Alzheimer's diseases. For example, many people develop trembling in their hands, have trouble walking, and feel weak.

Parkinson's Disease

Many people with advanced Parkinson's disease will develop dementia. Early signs of this type of dementia are problems with reasoning and judgment. For example, a person with Parkinson's disease dementia might have trouble understanding visual information or remembering how to do simple daily tasks. They may even have confusing or frightening hallucinations.

This type of dementia can also cause a person to be irritable. Many people become depressed or paranoid as the disease progresses. Others have trouble speaking and might forget words or get lost during a conversation.

Frontotemporal Dementia

Frontotemporal dementia is a name used to describe several types of dementia, all with one thing in common: they affect the front and side parts of the brain, which are the areas that control language and behavior. It's also known as Pick's disease.

Frontotemporal dementia affects people as young as 45 years old. Although scientists don't know what causes it, it does run in families and people with it have mutations in certain genes, according to the Alzheimer's Society.

This dementia causes loss of inhibitions and motivation, as well as compulsive behavior. It also causes people to have problems with speech, including forgetting the meaning of common words.

Creutzfeldt-Jakob Disease

Creutzfeldt-Jakob disease (CJD) is one of the rarest forms of dementia. Only 1 in 1 million people are diagnosed with it every year, according to the Alzheimer's Association. CJD progresses very quickly, and people often die within a year of diagnosis.

Symptoms of CJD are similar to other forms of dementia. Some people experience agitation, while others suffer from depression. Confusion and loss of memory are also common. CJD affects the body as well, causing twitching and muscle stiffness.

Wernicke-Korsakoff Syndrome

Wernicke's disease, or Wernicke's encephalopathy, is a type of brain disorder that's caused by a lack of vitamin B-1, leading to bleeding in the lower sections of the brain. Wernicke's disease can cause physical symptoms like double vision and a loss of muscle coordination. At a certain point, the physical symptoms of untreated Wernicke's disease tend to decrease, and the signs of Korsakoff syndrome start to appear.

Korsakoff syndrome is a memory disorder caused by advanced Wernicke's disease. People with Korsakoff syndrome may have trouble:

- processing information
- learning new skills
- remembering things

The two conditions are linked and usually grouped as one condition, known as Wernicke-Korsakoff syndrome. It's technically not a form of dementia. However, symptoms are similar to dementia, so it's often classified as such.

Wernicke-Korsakoff syndrome can be a result of malnutrition or chronic infections but, alcoholism and vitamin B1 deficiencies are the most common causes.

Sometimes, people with Wernicke-Korsakoff syndrome make up information to fill in the gaps in their memories without realizing what they're doing.

Mixed Dementia

Mixed dementia refers to a situation where a person has more than one type of dementia, which is very common. The most common combination is vascular dementia and Alzheimer's. According to the Jersey Alzheimer's Association, up to 45 percent of people with dementia have mixed dementia but don't know it.

Mixed dementia can cause different symptoms in different people. Some people experience memory loss and disorientation first, while others have behavior and mood changes. As the disease progresses, most people will have difficulty speaking and walking.

Normal Pressure Hydrocephalus

Normal Pressure Hydrocephalus (NPH) is a condition that causes a person to build up excess fluid in the brain's ventricles. The ventricles are fluid-filled spaces designed to cushion a person's brain and spinal cord. They rely on just the right amount of fluid to work properly. When the fluid builds up excessively, it places extra pressure on the brain. This can cause damage that leads to dementia symptoms. According to Johns Hopkins Medicine, an estimated 5 percent of dementia cases are due to NPH.

Huntington's Disease

Huntington's disease is a genetic condition that causes dementia. Two types exist: juvenile and adult-onset. The juvenile form is rarer and causes symptoms in childhood or adolescence. The adult form typically first causes symptoms in a person when they're in their 30s or 40s. The condition causes a premature breakdown of the brain's nerve cells, which can lead to dementia as well as impaired movement.

Other Causes of Dementia

Many diseases can cause dementia in later stages. For example, people with multiple sclerosis can develop dementia. It's also possible for those with HIV to develop cognitive impairment and dementia, especially if they're not taking antiviral medications.

FOOD FOR THOUGHT

Now that you are armed with some staggering yet enlightening information to help comprehend what dementia is about and how it affects people, do not be disheartened. Until there is a cure, there is care. Always remember there is a loving person still inside, and with continued training, knowledge, and self-awareness, you can help bring them out.

Chapter 2

More Good News...

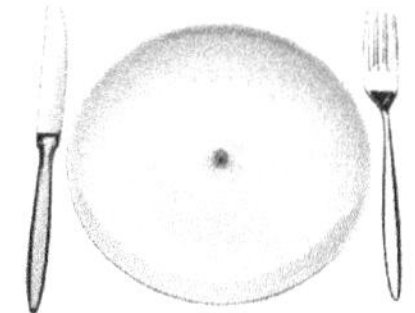

We have all been impacted by COVID-19, both professionally and personally. The presence of the virus has also created some significant challenges for those working with and living with dementia, especially those living in memory care or long-term care communities.

There is a common misunderstanding that individuals living with dementia cannot practice social distancing, which may result in their continued unnecessary and harmful isolation; fear not and think out of the box. There have been a lot of great ideas and practices put into place across the globe on how to balance the virus and isolation.

Individuals with dementia have the same needs as everyone else—to feel heard, cared for, safe, valued, and respected. As dementia progresses in the brain, memories of facts and skills for complex thought may fade, but feelings such as happiness, love, frustration, and sensing respect remain strong.

I have provided a bonus for you at the end of the book, a free pdf that will provide Five Sure-Fire Tips to Boost Communications During Covid-19 and Beyond.

FIVE COMMON CHALLENGES AND MISUNDERSTANDINGS

Let's focus on the following common challenges and misunderstandings about PLwD (People Living with Dementia) that may result in unnecessary and harmful isolation during these challenging times, particularly in a skilled nursing facility or other types of care/group communities.

1. It's impossible to keep people living with dementia 6 feet apart, so it's safer to keep them in their rooms all day.

- Allowing safe freedom of movement within the care community is essential. Everyone should have the opportunity to move about as freely as possible, but changes in the brain caused by dementia may mean that individuals are not able to exercise the judgment and reasoning to do it safely by maintaining a physical distance and wearing a mask. There are a number of reasons why a person with dementia needs to walk about, such as the need to engage in a familiar routine, desire to find the bathroom, want of exercise, or desire to relieve boredom.

- Do not try to keep the person seated all day in order to stop the walking about. This may cause anxiety, boredom, incontinence, poor circulation, constipation, and overall weakness, thus increasing the risk for falls. Walking helps elders maintain balance, gross motor skills, and overall healthy functioning of the body's systems. Could you bear sitting in a chair all day, every day? I don't think so.

- Getting to know your PLwD. If your loved one is in a facility, please communicate with the staff so they can get to know their routine and activities that will help keep them engaged and meet his or her needs. You should share what you know about your loved one and their past and present habits with the facility staff to anticipate or figure out why they feel compelled to walk about.

- Pay attention to when the desire to walk about occurs. It is common for an increase in noise to cause the person to want to get up and leave the area. Activity or noise that used to be easily tolerated or enjoyed, such as the TV, radio, or staff coming and going at shift change may now be overstimulating and uncomfortable. At home, it may be the grandkids running in and out of the house, dogs barking at deliveries, fire trucks, police cars, or heavy equipment vehicles that make a lot of noise as they drive by. Knowing the loud busy times is important so you can get PLwD to a quieter area of the house during those times.

- Ask the physician to help determine if the person is in pain, has a urinary tract infection, or is experiencing side effects of medications. PLwD oftentimes cannot recognize or express where the pain is coming from, so these unmet needs will express themselves through agitation.

- Create routines that involve movement. Suggest a daily walk. Accompanying the person at a safe distance on a daily walk or enlisting the help of family, friends, or volunteers to walk in a safe location, such as a courtyard, is a simple solution that usually works very well. Build this into the daily routine. Look for indoor opportunities in well-ventilated areas for regular exercises, such as an exercise class with a limited number of participants or seated exercises done with a video or internet-based tutorial.

- Many people walkabout out of boredom or because they are looking for something meaningful to do. If the person enjoys a certain type of hobby, try setting up a hobby table in their room where they can go and work on a project whenever they like. Provide cleaning materials such as a broom, dustpan and dusting cloths and invite the person to clean his or her room daily to encourage movement and purposeful activity. Social behaviors and the need to feel useful will always be a prevalent characteristic—embrace it.

- Try to encourage a healthy sleep routine for the person and avoid napping during the day, particularly due to lack of things to do. Provide orientation information such as the time of day. People with dementia often wake throughout the night and become confused about time. They may wake up in the middle of the night and get dressed. Having a large digital clock that shows AM and PM may help with the time confusion. Leaving a light on in the bathroom and the hallway may also help reduce disorientation at night. Avoiding daytime napping and spending time outdoors will also help encourage normal sleep patterns.

2. People with dementia will never remember to wash their hands or keep surfaces sanitized.

- Folks living with dementia will find it difficult to understand health information and remember to follow infection control guidance like washing their hands or wearing masks. It's our job to assist and set an example to protect all of our elders against COVID-19 or other instances of cross-contamination.

- If they ask (and they will repeatedly) why everyone is wearing a mask or why they must wear a mask, you can simply tell them there is a virus like the flu going around and everyone is trying to stay safe. Keep it simple, short, and don't offer too much detail, then redirect.

- Consider how much information to convey about COVID-19 to avoid inducing anxiety. Provide simple, basic information that is easy to understand for a person with cognitive impairment in a large print type size that is easy for elders with visual impairment to read. Encourage the elder to talk about any fears or concerns. Listen, reassure, comfort, and try to maintain a positive attitude. In this case, less is more, so keep the TV tuned to positive channels.

- Help elders make frequent handwashing part of the regular routine. Create positive visual reminders such as signs for the bathroom that state, "Clean hands feel good." Provide an essential oil scented warm cloth at each meal to use prior to eating and after the meal. Provide encouragement and celebrate accomplishments when the elder remembers to wash his or her hands. Make tissues, garbage cans, and sanitizer visually accessible throughout the community for easy access and a visual reminder to use them.

- Here is a gentle reminder...people with dementia often become confused when there are many steps in a sequence. You and I may not think that there are very many steps in the sequence of washing your hands, but there is a minimum of 12 steps to wash your hands:
    1. Walk to the sink.
    2. Figure out which handle is the cold water.
    3. Turn the handle to the right.
    4. Put your hands under the water to wet them.
    5. Find out where the soap is and how to use it.
    6. Press the soap pump or pick up the soap.
    7. Rub the soap between your hands.
    8. Rinse your hands under the water.
    9. Turn the water off by finding the correct handle again and turn it to the left.
    10. Find a towel.
    11. Dry your hands with a towel and dispose of it in the trash or rehang on a towel rod.
    12. Exit the restroom without touching the doorknob and contaminating your hands.

Think about all the common tasks we complete every single day. We shower, make our bed, get dressed, fix our meals, etc. Each one of these tasks has multiple steps. A person with dementia can experience a breakdown or lapse in sequence during any of these steps. When you notice someone having trouble with something you think is simple, pause for a moment, be patient, try to figure out which step caused trouble or confusion and help them through it.

3. People cannot effectively communicate with someone with dementia while wearing a mask.

- If you can do so with or without a face shield, enter the room, and greet the person living with dementia. Once a connection is established, use this opportunity to demonstrate putting on your mask properly, thus encouraging the elder to copy your actions and don theirs.

- Help PLwD make mask-wearing part of the regular routine. After their morning routine, suggest placing a mask on one's face before leaving the room.

- Provide a hook for the mask with a large reminder note inside the bedroom or near the door as a reminder to put on a mask before exiting.

- Provide staff or family members with a positive statement (mantra) about using masks that each person uses to communicate the same positive message.

- Remove masks prior to entering an elder's room to greet the person at a physical distance and allow the person to see the face of the staff or family member.

- Wear high contrast large print name tags with your first name only and a large, clear photo of yourself. Place the tag on the chest area, always in the same spot so it can be clearly seen.

- Always look the person in the eye when communicating, especially with a mask on. Use positive gestures and maintain a calm presence.

4. It's hard to keep someone with cognitive impairment engaged in something for very long.

- People can sociably distance by engaging with different personalized activities at tables that are a safe distance apart, in their rooms with the door open, or in small group activities in well-ventilated areas. A small worktable with projects of interest can relieve boredom and decrease anxiety.

- Consider a schedule during which different people walk throughout the hall at different times of the day; establishing a routine of movement while reducing the number of people in the halls at one time, respecting the need for social distancing. Do not discount purposeful activities, such as working indoors or outdoors by cleaning, planting, or weeding of plants/flowers and vegetable/herb gardens. These activities can add to a sense of routine and can be a good way to socialize.

- People with dementia can learn new routines and can follow written cues, gestures, and demonstrations by others. PATIENCE! A care partner can invite them to participate in an activity, demonstrate the process with their hands positioned so that they can see them clearly and move at a steady, unhurried pace. This would allow your loved one to understand how to complete the activity and be independent, engaging with the materials themselves.

5. Keeping families safely connected with their loved ones.

The social and emotional well-being of both family members and elders is often centered around maintaining frequent contact with one another. Because of the physical distance required during COVID-19, families are concerned about their loved one's health. In addition, both parties can experience anxiety and loneliness from the separation. Stay alert to the latest guidelines set forth by governing regulatory authorities in your area.

- Staff can be asked to assist elders and families with regular visual access to their loved ones by setting up recurring appointments for video conferencing or connecting with their loved ones routinely by phone.

- Staff can be asked to assist elders in writing letters, cards, or emails to family and friends. Provide cards, stationery, and stamps and invite the elder to dictate a letter (or email).

- Staff may suggest that families create a memory box or care package with a variety of interesting items such as photos, travel memorabilia, trinkets, favorite snacks, or magazines for the elder to enjoy. It would be helpful for family and staff to share the meaning or value of the memorabilia.

- Family visits should be limited to two people at a time. Family members should follow the community protocol for masks, handwashing and the use of sanitizer upon entering the building. Whenever possible, the use of name tags should be utilized to assist PLwD with name recognition. A variety of visiting space options should be provided in areas that can be ventilated by opening windows. Outdoor space should also have chairs properly spaced apart for social distancing.

- A variety of activity ideas should be available for families to enjoy together, such as gardening, listening to music, playing games, taking walks, or filling bird feeders.

- Personalized materials can be provided and kept in individuals' rooms, so they are always available. Other materials that are sanitized after use can be made available on tables throughout different areas of the community. A variety of kits can be assembled with supplies and given to elders who express interest in the topic.

In summary, when this pandemic ends, we will likely still be faced with some variant of social distancing. The precautions we are required to practice today in order to prevent the spread of contaminants may, unfortunately, become the norm in high-risk, compromised communities, such as a skilled nursing facility or group community.

Please bear in mind that many individuals living with dementia can practice safe social distancing with the appropriate person-centered care practices and procedures in place. This statement bears repeating: individuals with dementia have the same needs as everyone else—to feel heard, cared for, safe, valued, and respected. This is especially important now as states move to partially reopen care communities to visitors when social distancing can be practiced.

FOOD FOR THOUGHT

Everyone is a unique individual and in turn, responds differently to distinctive stimulations. The more you know about the likes/dislikes and habits of PLwD in your care, the better you can serve them and serve yourself. In the absence of a cure for dementia, socialization and engagement in purposeful activities are a powerful treatment for the symptoms associated with dementia.

PLwD still need to feel wanted, learn new information, have relationships with friends and family, and contribute to the community. Social isolation because of COVID-19 puts PLwD at risk for decline in mental and physical functioning, loneliness, and depression. Think outside the box and use all the resources available to you through the internet, your peers, and professional organizations

Chapter 3

Why Won't Mom Eat or Drink?

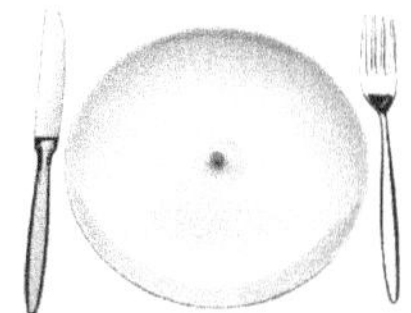

Is My Loved One Suffering?

As a care partner, the most important concern is that the person with dementia does not suffer. Once we understand the normal progression of the disease, it makes it easier to see why PLwD do not need as much to eat or drink.

The body of a person who has a life-limiting illness is in the process of shutting down. They no longer require a great deal of nutrients or calories to convert to energy and therefore, their appetite or desire for food diminishes. A person at the end of their life does not experience or show signs of hunger or thirst in the way a healthy person does.

A balanced diet is preferable, but not so important as the disease progresses into the later stages and end of life. Consult with your registered dietitian but consider offering the person foods and drinks that they appear to be able to swallow and are desirable foods they have preferred in the past. Generally speaking, it is fine to honor these requests unless there have been severe restrictions placed on the person's nutrition plan. If they want only sweet things or cold things, accommodate them.

Put on Your Detective Hat!

Eating and drinking is a complex process that involves the control center in the brain and strong muscles in the neck and throat. As dementia progresses, it affects these areas, which then expresses as symptoms that the care partner sees, such as coughing or choking, clearing the throat, grimacing when swallowing, exaggerated movements of the mouth or tongue, refusal to swallow, holding food in the mouth, or spitting food out.

First, rule out any physical problems such as mouth sores, a toothache, ill-fitting dentures, infections, or medications that could be affecting appetite. Then, try changing the food or drinks offered. Give soft but flavorful food that requires minimal chewing and a variety of temperatures with each meal. Avoid hard foods, foods with stringy textures and mixed foods (liquids and solids combo) like cereal and chunky soups. Use smaller utensils and specially designed drinking cups. Have the person sit upright in a comfortable position. Allow extra time as it can take some extra effort but will be worth it as you see them enjoy a meal. If you observe choking, coughing or overall difficulties chewing and safely swallowing foods, seek professional attention from your physician or speech therapist for recommendations.

What Are Some Other Things I Should Know?

Don't forget, everyone is different and there is truly no cookie-cutter approach to engage effectively with PLwD, regardless of the stage or level of dementia they are in. A clinical study completed in Korea compared the swallowing problems of people with late-stage Alzheimer's to those with vascular dementia. Those with Alzheimer's had more trouble swallowing fluids, while those with vascular dementia struggled more with swallowing food.

It is also important to note the finding that those with frontotemporal dementia have links to behavior that affects their relationship with food. Some individuals may eat compulsively, eat only sweets, or will eat very quickly, shoving food into their mouths until they choke. Knowing these facts is important in discussions regarding how to proceed with caring for these different aspects of the disease. Work with the professionals who are supporting you and your loved one to discover what works best for your current situation and upcoming potential changes in consumption.

Disclaimer: Please be aware that the above is merely informational—**not medical advice**. If you need medical advice, please consult your doctor or other appropriate healthcare professionals.

30 Reasons PLwD Might Decline to Eat

People with dementia are PEOPLE. Regarding the situation of refusing to eat, read the responses below and you may change your mind and proclaim that their behavior is "NORMAL." Ask yourself why you might refuse food, and you will likely have the answer to the question of why someone with dementia might decline to eat.

Here is a list of 30 potential reasons someone living with dementia (or someone NOT living with dementia for that matter) might decline to eat:

1. He/she is not hungry.

2. He/she doesn't care for the food they are being offered.

3. He/she doesn't like the way the food is presented (e.g. the color, the texture, the fact that it's pureed or not, or it doesn't even LOOK like food).

4. He/she doesn't like the smell of the food.

5. He/she doesn't like the taste of the food or the food tastes bad.

6. The food is too hot or too cold.

7. He/she is sick.

8. He/she is tired and doesn't feel like eating.

9. He/she is in pain.

10. His or her tummy is upset or they have cramps.

11. He/she is having trouble swallowing and is afraid they might choke.

12. He/she is sedated with drugs that they're not interested in eating or physically can't eat.

13. He/she doesn't remember how to use the utensils and doesn't want to be impolite by using their hands.

14. It's not their usual mealtime as it's too early or too late.

15. Someone is telling them/ giving them an order to eat and they hate people telling them what to do.

16. Someone is trying to feed him/her when they are perfectly capable of feeding themselves.

17. He/she needs help to eat but is too afraid to ask for help or there's no one around to help.

18. It's too noisy / it's too quiet.

19. He/she is tired of eating the same thing all the time.

20. The place he/she is in is unfamiliar. They prefer to eat where they usually eat.

21. He/she prefers to eat what they want and no one asked what they wanted.

22. The lights are too bright / the lights are too dim.

23. He/she feels constipated / needs to go to the bathroom.

24. He/she is surrounded by strange people and wants to go home and eat with their family.

25. He/she wants to sit with their friend at another table but is not "allowed" to.

26. His/her dentures don't fit properly and it's hard for them to chew.

27. He/she doesn't seem to have their dentures anymore, and can't eat properly without them.

28. Whenever he/she eats, they get some kind of adverse reaction, so they're refusing to eat to avoid the reaction.

29. He/she saw someone crush pills into their food, and doesn't want to take the pills.

30. He/she is at the end of life and just doesn't feel like eating anymore.

FOOD FOR THOUGHT

No doubt there are other reasons not noted, but the important thing to remember is that people who live with dementia are just like the rest of us. They are human beings with thoughts, feelings, needs, likes, and dislikes.

If we took the time to step back and ask ourselves about why people who live with dementia react as they do, who or what may have triggered that reaction, we would be better able to serve them and in turn, serve ourselves.

Chapter 4

Ringing the Dinner Bell

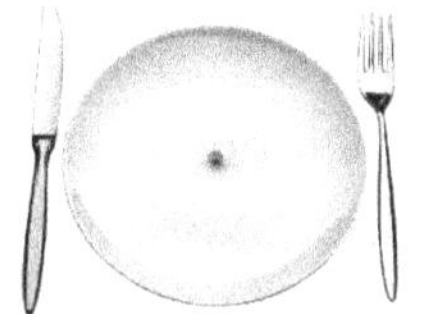

Your Model Dining Area

We all know mealtimes are an opportunity to boost satisfaction and quality of life, but for People Living with Dementia (PLwD), there are often additional concerns to address. It's important for PLwD to stay focused and free from agitation long enough to receive adequate nutrition while ensuring a positive and social dining experience.

Four Steps to Enhancing the Dining Experience

Here are four broad categories, and some commonsense solutions to help improve the overall dining experience for PLwD.

1. Atmosphere: Soothe Anxiety

Create a dementia-friendly environment by using memory aids to remind PLwD about mealtimes. Try a clock with large numbers, an easy-to-read appointment calendar with large letters and numbers, or even a daily schedule wipe-off board in their room, or a menu board easily accessible in a high traffic or common area.

Aromatherapy is well known and used throughout our own homes and many memory care communities, not only for mealtimes, but to enhance the living space ambiance throughout the day as well. Start the day off by diffusing a citrus or mint blend to pep up the person living with dementia as they begin their day (you will appreciate the benefits yourself too). Another easy and pleasant tip is to use infused (and warmed) hand wipes or towels prior to meal service; use lemon or orange essential oil to lightly scent the moist hand towel. Change it up for the dinner meal and diffuse lavender to bring about calm to the mealtime.

Here is a word of advice regarding essential oils. Always take the time to check the labels on your essential oils and be sure they are therapeutic grade. An easy way to check this for off-the-shelf products (other than the impulsive, wow that's inexpensive/cheap) is if the label says, "Do not apply to skin," then you probably shouldn't breathe or diffuse it either! Go for the good stuff, a few drops of quality therapeutic grade oil will go a long way to meet your needs.

The design of the dining space plays a significant impact on PLwD's challenges, while at the same time, improves the culture of the person-centered care philosophy. Once inside the dining space, be consistent with furniture placement so they know what to expect. The dining room should look like a dining room, not a workshop, media room, etc. You can play soothing music (but not too loud) for a calming effect while diffusing essential oils that will stimulate the appetite—try rosemary, ginger, or citrus. While making the dining space calm and relaxed, it is just as important to avoid overstimulation caused by television, excessive noises, or too many people moving about or talking and creating a distraction. This should be a social event where you are seated next to and engaging the person living with dementia while encouraging and monitoring food and beverage consumption for nutritional intake.

Let's not forget about the impact of lighting. Exposure to bright light has been studied as a non-pharmacological treatment for elderly people with Alzheimer's. A positive impact of light therapy on cognition was observed in various studies. They found PLwD exposed to bright light were more awake, and verbally competent. The well-being of PLwD has been measured by researchers and it was determined that exposure to bright light improved PLwD's moods. Sounds good to me! The added value is that brighter lights can improve seeing and help PLwD manage what they are doing as they engage their eating and drinking skills.

2. Tabletops: Keep it Simple

When caring for PLwD, keep the table setting basic, and only offer the utensils they will need. That also means avoiding patterned plates and tablecloths as well as minimizing decorations and condiments on the table that might cause unnecessary distraction.

However, creating contrast is still an important part of dining. Many PLwD suffer from visual impairment so the distinction between the food, the plate and tablecloth should be considered. For that, use brightly colored dinnerware, which will help PLwD identify where the food is on the plate.

In fact, a Boston University study found, "Older adults dining from red plates ate 25% more than those dining from white plates." The color red in itself is not the end-all answer, the point is that when you have white sliced turkey, beige potatoes and rutabagas on a white plate, set on a white table cover—the food is indistinguishable. Add diminished vision and PLwD simply cannot see the food.

Consideration for what PLwD eat with or on can also improve their overall dining experience. Remember, this is about them and their abilities and not your preferences. Increase their independence by substituting a bowl for a plate, a spoon for a fork, or choosing from assistive dinnerware, mugs and flatware that address some of the physical issues associated with aging. For example, large handles offer a more comfortable grip, weighted utensils keep things steady, coated utensils protect lips and teeth, and two-handed mugs with lids help reduce spills. More information on the topic of dinnerware and assisted feeding will be covered later in the book.

What about the table itself? At times, not much thought goes into selecting a table that is at the correct height to accommodate the need of PLwD who may be using a special needs chair, a custom-made dining room chair or a wheelchair. At times, when using tables with chairs that have taller arms, they are unable to push their chairs close enough to reach their place setting at the table, making it difficult for them to reach their meal. It can be frustrating when food on the table is out of reach for anyone, but for an elderly person or one suffering from dementia, this frustration can progress to annoyance and possibly cause them to refuse to eat at all. Think out of the box on this one—can you raise the table with blocks? Can they transfer from a wheelchair to a regular chair with arms? Can you lower the table or add a ramp to safely raise their wheelchair higher above the table lip? Get creative! PLwD need to be provided with every opportunity to feed themselves and get adequate nutrition.

3. Menus & Mealtime: Strategy is Important

PLwD are most alert and hungry in the morning, so either serve more food (high in nutrient value—not sugary fillers) at breakfast or serve several breakfasts. Be flexible with mealtimes and give plenty of time to eat without rushing. The time between ordering/choosing their food and getting the food should also be minimal—if the food takes too long to serve, PLwD may forget what they ordered or why they are even in the dining room and get frustrated.

Get those morning food smells going with aromas of coffee brewing, waffles/pancakes cooking (vanilla or cinnamon) or breakfast meats sizzling in the pan. Does this sound good to you? Well, it appeals to them too! Later in the day, other enticing aromas such as the smell of fresh-baked cookies, soups or breads will help to increase appetite as well.

In general, a dementia-friendly food menu should consist of smaller meals with just one or two food choices at a time, rather than three large, multi-course meals a day. Finger foods, like sandwiches, wraps and fresh fruit and vegetables, are ideal dementia-friendly food and should be incorporated into your meal and menu planning. This gives PLwD who have lost strength, coordination, or dexterity an opportunity to stay focused on eating instead of getting frustrated over the challenge of managing their flatware. You can even look at creative ways to transform familiar foods into finger foods.

Would you want to be seen juggling your food and spilling it on the table or yourself during a meal? What about hot beverages or soups? No one does and this can cause both physical and emotional pain in addition to embarrassment in front of their peers, so they just won't eat and say, "I'm not hungry." We will dive deeper into menu and food recommendations, and adaptive eating dishware and utensils in a later chapter.

4. Socialization: Get Involved

Just like anyone, feeling involved and part of the conversation can have a big emotional impact on PLwD. With that in mind, greet them sincerely and engage in conversation before, during and after meals—even if they are not able to respond verbally. When possible, sit and eat with them and offer assistance throughout the meal. Please do not confuse assistance with doing the task at hand for them. These folks can manage just fine if prompted appropriately. Just keep in mind that while others may be joining the meal, their focus should remain on our diner and not chit-chat amongst themselves as if PLwD are only objects in the space. Consider how you felt if you have ever been ignored or dismissed in a group setting. These folks are still with us but cannot necessarily express themselves.

For PLwD in the early stages of cognitive decline, family-style dining offers the chance to reminisce and socialize with each other, making dining a more engaging part of the day. When food will be eaten right away, use lightweight serving pieces to pass around (these dishes are not suited to holding temperatures, just as serving vessels). Increase the socialization by replacing institutional clothing protectors with, for example, attractive machine washable dinner wear, such as wearing dining scarves.

FOOD FOR THOUGHT

Where do I sit, where do I fit? Well, my dear loved one, you fit right in with the rest of the folks at the table. The family dinner table usually has Dad at the head of the table and Mom at the opposite end with kids and other family members filling in the circle. This pattern has gone on for umpteen years as family dynamics change, and Dad is still Dad, Mom is still Mom, except now they move a little slower and need a bit more attention. Who are we to deny them that position of respect? #dinewithdignity means just what it says.

A real challenge when caring for people with dementia is to get over ourselves and our agendas. The roles have been reversed and that's all there is to it—so embrace it and be there for your loved ones. So now, instead of Mom using salad & dinner forks, steak knives, 12" dinner plates and delicate crystal wine glasses, she eats (and feeds herself) utilizing a spoon, bowl and weighted mug. Who really has the problem here? Take a deep breath and utilize as many strategies specific to their capabilities to help improve their overall dining and food consumption experience.

Chapter 5

Ya Gotta Eat

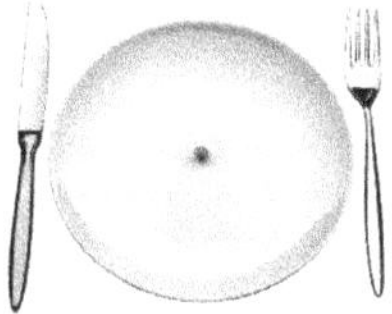

This chapter will provide basic, yet important information and tips as we dive into nutrition and hydration for People Living with Dementia (PLwD). Dysphagia (or difficulty swallowing) will be discussed here on an informational basis only. You can access tools to help you familiarize yourself with the recommended guidelines. This information is provided for your consideration and not medical advice; always seek out guidance from appropriate professionals, such as your speech therapist, registered dietitian, certified dietary manager, and physician.

Dysphagia Defined

Dysphagia (or difficulty swallowing) means it takes more time and effort to move food or liquid from your mouth to your stomach.

Dysphagia may also be associated with pain. In some cases, swallowing may be impossible.

Occasional difficulty swallowing, which may occur when you eat too fast or don't chew your food well enough, usually isn't cause for concern. But persistent dysphagia may indicate a serious medical condition requiring treatment. Chewing is not only an important part of the digestive process, but it's also beneficial to overall health. People who don't chew their food well enough before they swallow often develop digestive problems and are also at a greater risk for choking.

Dysphagia may lead to aspiration. Aspiration is when something enters your airway or lungs by accident. It may be food, liquid, or some other material. This can cause serious health problems, such as pneumonia. Aspiration can happen when you have trouble swallowing normally. Dysphagia can occur at any age, but it's more common in older adults. The cause of swallowing problems vary, and treatment depends on the cause. As PLwD progress in their stage of dementia, you should have them assessed by appropriate medical experts. In the case of dysphagia, a speech therapist and registered dietitian should be consulted.

Care Partner Tips: Nutrition and Hydration

As we age, the need for a balanced diet becomes more important. Ensuring adequate nutrition and hydration may be more difficult for those living with dementia. There are several reasons that could lead to a deficit in nutrition and hydration for these individuals, but there are also helpful hints and possibilities to make nutrition and hydration an easier venture.

Timing of Medication Administration

- Often, those living with dementia are suspicious or skeptical about medications given to them. They may develop a mistrust of the person offering the medication and refuse to take it. If these medications are given at mealtime, the medication refusal may cause the meal to be refused as well. Not good!

- Some medications are to be taken with meals; set them aside until after the meal so the medication struggle isn't part of mealtime.

- Clear all evidence of the meal and then offer the medication.

- Sometimes, you can relieve many of the issues by eliminating taking oral medications. Utilizing other medication types, such as liquid medication, patches or inhaled medication, may yield benefits. Ask your physician or pharmacist if this is an option.

- New medications may alter or decrease appetite. Monitor them closely and notify a physician if there is a significant change. You should always ask questions about any medications that your loved one is taking; the why, the dosage and the possible side effects.

Issues of the Mouth

- There may be pain related to eating for a person living with dementia. They may or may not be able to communicate this to you. They could have overly dry and cracked lips, canker sores, loose or broken teeth, sensitivity to food temperatures, or cheek or tongue cuts and abrasions—take the time to look if they are demonstrating pain.

- Dentures that don't fit well may cause difficulty with chewing and make it uncomfortable to eat. It is important to visit the dentist on a regular basis to ensure any issues with teeth and gums are addressed.

- Some people living with dementia will complain about sensitivity around the mouth area that makes it uncomfortable to eat or drink. Do not dismiss this; take the time to investigate their concerns and take appropriate action. Remember that they may not be able to express themselves clearly and indicate where the pain originates.

- Offer a warm and soft cloth to wash and wipe the mouth area before eating. Often, stimulating the mouth area with a cloth is beneficial to prepare for eating.

- For some, brushing their teeth is beneficial before a meal. Offer this option as well, but be sure to rinse well if you are doing this before the meal—no one wants peppermint flavor mixing with drinks or foods.

- Always test the food being served to ensure that the temperature is not too hot or too cold.

Appetite Changes, Taste, and Smell

- With all the sensory and cognitive changes a person living with dementia experiences, you should expect that your loved one may experience changes in appetite and food preferences.

- Foods they have loved for decades may now have a negative smell or taste. Don't force these foods or argue over them. They may not remember that a certain food was a favorite and only know that it smells or tastes bad now.

- Offer a variety of balanced foods: vegetables, fruits, whole grains, low-fat dairy products, and lean proteins.

- Offer small servings at first until you understand new preferences and realize they may change again. Offer no more than two choices at once. For example: something cold or hot to drink? Vegetables or fruit? Too many choices will confuse PLwD and cause anxiety.

- Depending on the cognitive impairment of your loved one, they may not recognize the food or know what to do with it. Be patient.

- You may need to demonstrate picking up the food and eating it. Sometimes, people living with dementia need help getting started on a task.

- A visual demonstration is best for understanding.

Distractions at Mealtime

- Offer a calm environment for mealtime; too much activity or interaction can be difficult for a person living with dementia to stay focused on eating the meal.

- Remove other objects from the table or food tray.
- If possible, turn the television off during the meal.
- Sit with the person who is eating, even if you are not. You don't have to talk, but it may be calming to have someone sitting nearby and not standing or looming over them.
- If mealtime is more of a social event for family to gather, your loved one may enjoy it more and be more willing to eat and drink.
- Arrange food on a plate that is a contrasting color; otherwise, visual changes may cause the person living with dementia to have trouble seeing the difference between the food and the plate.
- Be cognizant of their field of vision; as dementia progresses, they go from full field vision to binocular and then to monocular vision. Observe if they are only focusing on certain quadrants at the table and move or adjust the dish and glassware.
- Give the person living with dementia plenty of time to eat. It may take over an hour for your loved one to eat the entire meal. Encourage independence by letting them finish their meal on their own if they can do so safely.

Utensils, Chewing and Choking

- There may be times when your loved one cannot recall how to use a utensil. You can visually demonstrate usage, which may prompt them to use a spoon or fork. You may need to put the utensil in their hand.
- Consider changing the service ware to meet the needs of your loved one. For example, bowls or plates with raised edges for scooping and the use of spoons versus forks.
- To ensure safety, you may want to offer meals cut into finger food sizes so that your loved one can feed themself, either with a utensil or by hand.
- Promoting independence is vital, so eating with your hands should always be acceptable.
- Avoid foods that require thorough chewing as this may prove difficult for those living with dementia. Some examples of foods that require thorough chewing are steaks, pork chops and raw carrots.
- Pocketing portions of food in the sides of the mouth might occur if your loved one cannot get it all chewed up and swallowed. This will eventually become a choking hazard.
- At some point, you might find it beneficial to serve ground, minced and moist, or pureed foods to ensure they can be swallowed safely. Seek out a speech therapist who can conduct an evaluation to determine what consistency of food is best suited and appropriate for your loved one.

- Generally speaking, if you have concerns about choking due to chewing challenges, start with some softer foods such as cottage cheese, yogurt, applesauce, or scrambled eggs. Contact your medical team and let them know if you are observing a pattern of choking or difficulty swallowing, they can guide you to appropriate steps to take to ensure your loved one's safety and well-being.

- Regardless of whether your loved one is at home with you or living in a community, learn the Heimlich maneuver so you are prepared to provide assistance in the event of choking.

Hydration

- Lack of hydration is a big problem for those living with dementia. Encourage and offer liquids often. Get and keep easily identifiable covered water cups/containers accessible in different rooms of the house as visual cues.

- Prompt fluid intake by having a drink along with your loved one. Modeling behavior is a good way to encourage intake.

- Sometimes, there is a fear of drinking water, typically related to a fear of choking. Use a dark-colored drinking cup and enhance plain water with a splash of fresh fruit juice or single drops of lemon, orange, or lime therapeutic grade essential oils.

- Offer hot or cold drinks. Sometimes, coffee is a great way to start the day. You might find that your loved one prefers room temperature drinks instead of ice-cold. With the mouth sensitivity, cold may be too uncomfortable and they may no longer want any ice in their beverages.

- Urinary tract infections are a big concern, so pushing fluids is important. With this comes the need to regularly go to the toilet, so have a plan and a routine to maintain sanitary conditions and dignity.

- Offer foods that have a high water content as well. Some choices are celery, berries, melons, cucumbers, apples, clear soups, or broth. Be aware of their chewing capabilities to prevent opportunities for choking.

Problem Food and Drinks

Certain foods may cause problems for your loved one, so if they are experiencing any issues, these could be the culprits:

- Caffeine
- Grapefruit (interaction with certain medications)
- Meats (pork, poultry, beef)
- Cheese or milk
- Fatty foods
- Salt
- Sugar
- Diet drinks

Always consult and engage your physician in helping you determine next steps in appropriate care.

Interventions

Some Useful Mealtime Strategies for PLwD:

- If the dining area is used for multiple activities, offer distinct environmental cues to signal the change from a recreational activity to eating
- Increase lighting and contrast at the table setting
- Use visual cues and written reminders
- Control noise, light glare, and odor
- Serve promptly after they are seated
- Offer visual cues for boundaries by using place mats or square tables to reduce interest in another's meal
- Decorate the dining room in a homelike manner to provide reassurance and environmental cues
- Supervise the meal, cue, and encourage eating, use one-step directives
- Limit the number of utensils (usually people will choose the utensil closest to their dominant hand)
- Use cups with large enough handles that are easy to grasp
- Serving larger portions for breakfast may help to maintain weight

- Increase the number of finger foods and provide foods "on the go"

- PLwD can often be tempted to eat by adding sweeteners or other such seasonings to food; be sure to monitor the condiments that are left in the open for usage—it is best to limit access

- Serve one item at a time to decrease distractions and limit choices

- Provide ethnic or culturally appropriate foods

- Alternate hot and cold, add sweetener, and alternate with spicy foods, add ketchup, mustard, or salt and pepper (if medically appropriate)

- Tell concerned individuals that their meals are paid for, provide meal tickets or imitation money, or explain that it is included in a meal club

- Offer liquids and water consistently throughout the day and have access to beverage stations throughout frequently traveled areas

- Repeat redirection to the task of eating meals and snacks

- Do not use garnishes or decorations that are not easily chewed

- Make a small table for one or two if they perform better when eating alone or in a small group

Nutrition and Standards

Diet and nutrition play an important role in maintaining health and well-being. You are, after all, what you eat. Diet can be defined as what we habitually eat and drink. Diet is thus best conceived as a lifestyle and plays a relevant role in both morbidity and mortality. This next section will have information for your own knowledge regarding nutrition, eating, and weight loss. Let me note that some of the comments and activities will refer specifically to what takes place either in a skilled nursing facility or group community—which is good for you to know also.

Nutrition can be simply defined as the use of foods that humans (and all living organisms) make to live and maintain their health. Nutrition encompasses the processes of ingesting and digesting foods and absorbing and metabolizing their nutrients. It is implicated in the provision of water, micronutrients (i.e., vitamins and minerals), macronutrients (i.e., carbohydrates, proteins, and lipids), and energy.

These components are used by the human body to build and maintain tissues, and to allow its optimal functioning, hence adequate nutrition is essential for healthy living. Malnutrition comprises both overnutrition (excess food/calorie intake) and undernutrition, which is the depletion of body energy stores and loss of body mass (mainly lean mass).

Malnutrition results mainly from eating an inadequate diet in which the quantity and/or quality of nutrients does not meet the needs of our body. Health status influences diet, and several diseases may concomitantly lead to excess losses of micronutrients and increased energy expenditure, which can also cause and exacerbate malnutrition.

According to the Alzheimer's Association UK, undernutrition (insufficient calories, protein or other nutrients needed for tissue maintenance and repair) is the most common nutritional problem, affecting up to 10% of older people living at home, 30% of those living in care homes, and 70% of hospitalized older people.

Nutritional standards of care for people with dementia should be introduced throughout the health and social care sectors and monitored for compliance. While weight loss is a common problem for people with dementia, undernutrition can and should be avoided. Proof of concept comes from a review of the use of oral nutritional supplements, such as Ensure, indicating that it is possible to stabilize or even increase the weight of people with dementia over relatively long periods.

Understanding Weight Loss in Advanced Dementia

Studies have shown that once dementia reaches its final stages, one in every two or three affected people will experience severe weight loss. Weight loss may occur despite the person with advanced dementia being given all the food they want. Weight loss may be part of the process of dying from dementia. Watching someone with advanced dementia lose weight, despite being fed enough food, can be frightening. It is quite normal to feel this way. Staff in the facility will talk to you about any weight loss issues your family member/friend is facing and support you as you make decisions relating to their care.

How is Weight Loss Monitored?

Staff monitor and document weight loss by regularly weighing every person with advanced dementia. If they are losing weight or having problems eating, staff monitor them every week while the problems persist. Sometimes they stop weighing residents with advanced dementia, even though they know they are losing weight as being weighed will disturb them and the main goal is to keep them as comfortable as possible. Staff should only stop weighing PLwD after the family members, general practitioner and facility staff have discussed it and agreed that it is no longer appropriate.

What Changes in Weight Are Looked Out For?

Family members and medical staff should particularly watch out for anyone who has:

- A five percent weight loss in one month. For example, a person who weighs 150 lb. and loses 7.5 lb. in one month will be monitored carefully.

- Less appetite than usual. Everyone's appetite can change, especially when starting a new medication or just being ill. If a poor appetite continues, we need to consider the cause.

- A slow decrease in the amount of body fat so they are underweight for their height.

- Unexpected weight loss for three consecutive months. Weight, like appetite, can fluctuate without there being a problem. Unexpected weight loss that continues for three months, however, needs to be investigated further.

- If you are caring for your loved one at home, and identify decreased consumption of food and liquids, contact your medical team and seek direction on next steps. It is better to ask before the results have a serious negative impact on their health.

What Are Some Common Reasons For Weight Loss?

- Not eating enough food. In this case, you should look at the food given to the PLwD to see whether it needs to be changed. They might not like the food or it could be the wrong consistency and they are having trouble swallowing it. They might need a larger serving. A dietitian or speech pathologist may need to be engaged to investigate.

- Your loved one might not be eating enough because they have bad teeth, poorly fitting dentures, or mouth ulcers. They may need to see a dentist or have their daily mouth care changed so they are more comfortable. Remember, PLwD may not be able to communicate the location or type of pain they are experiencing. We are the ones that must pay attention to changes, such as noticing they started chewing on one side only, and take action to investigate.

- We should also consider how much help each person needs to eat a meal and, if necessary, give them more help. Consider how they are physically "arranged" during mealtime, especially if they are sitting in a Geri Chair or are bed-bound.

Are they slumped over and not sitting upright? Can they comfortably reach and access the food components on the tray and bedside table? Are the food containers sealed and difficult to open on their own (fruit cups, juice, jellos)? Is there a giant hideous dome covering the plate and they don't know what steps to take next (remember they have dementia—never assume). Think about it, visualize the situations I'm describing from their perspective.

What Types of Medical Problems May Cause Weight Loss?

Some conditions can be managed so weight loss slows down or stops, such as:

- Depression
- Constipation
- Pain
- Some medications
- Thyroid disease
- Chronic infections
- Special diets such as low cholesterol diets
- Not drinking enough fluids

Sometimes blood tests, X-rays or other medical tests are needed to confirm these conditions. Invasive tests, such as taking blood, may disturb a person with advanced dementia. It is important to consider whether knowing the test result is more important than disturbing the person. You may decide that you no longer want your loved one to have any more invasive tests. Staff will support whatever decision you make. For many frail people with advanced dementia, this may be the most appropriate choice.

What Can be Done When the Weight Loss Continues?

Weight loss may continue even though the common reasons for weight loss have been managed. Weight loss can be inevitable due to an advanced disease called cachexia (ka/kek/sia). Cachexia is a normal process caused by advanced diseases such as dementia and cancer, heart, liver, kidney, or lung failure. When people have cachexia, they can't absorb the nutrients from food, even when they are eating and drinking enough. They lose weight, have no appetite, and become tired and weak. The person's body slows down and prepares for death.

What can be done about continued weight loss? When cachexia is present, the best choice is to carefully feed the person using food he/she likes and can safely swallow. This way, the person can still enjoy the social contact that comes from eating. Tastes and smells from favorite foods can stimulate the appetite. Family members and friends can help feed the person if they want to help. A person with cachexia should never be forced to eat.

What is Artificial Tube Feeding?

Sometimes feeding tubes are considered. These tubes are inserted directly into the stomach to artificially feed a person who has trouble eating or swallowing. Feeding tubes stop the person from enjoying the social contact of being fed and the taste of foods they like. Feeding tubes are not normally recommended for people with advanced dementia, as they are uncomfortable and may cause infections or bleeding where they are inserted.

Research shows that being fed through a feeding tube does not help a person live longer than if they were carefully fed their favorite foods. If artificial feeding via a tube commences, it may need to be stopped as vomiting or breathlessness from having extra fluid in the body might make dying more uncomfortable. The decision to stop tube feeding is sometimes harder to make than the decision to start it.

Making Decisions is Hard!

Food is a very important part of our lives. We cook food for others to show our love for them. We eat special food at celebrations such as birthdays and weddings. We enjoy social contact as we share food. Having to make decisions about feeding and weight loss is hard. When a person has advanced dementia and can't tell us what they want, it's even harder. Think about what your family member would want and base your decisions on that. Talk to the nurses and other staff in the facility and the general practitioner, who knows your loved one well. They all want them to be comfortable and honored. If you remain very worried, consider speaking to your spiritual advisor or a close friend about the issues to gain extra support.

Note: in a skilled care setting, there should be scheduled care plan meetings engaging you where you can ask specific questions regarding the care your family member is receiving. The community where your loved one is living must respond to your inquiries in a timely fashion—don't hesitate to ask your questions and get answers. You have the right to ask questions about their care programs.

MyPlate for Older Adults

MyPlate for Older Adults is based on the 2015-2020 Dietary Guidelines for Americans. Most guidelines apply to adults of any age, while the new MyPlate offers adjustments to meet the needs of older Americans.

MyPlate for Older Adults
Fruits & Vegetables
Whole fruits and vegetables are rich in important nutrients and fiber. Choose fruits and vegetables with deeply colored flesh. Choose canned varieties that are packed in their own juices or low-sodium.
Healthy Oils
Liquid vegetable oils and soft margarines provide important fatty acids and some fat-soluble vitamins.
Herbs & Spices
Use a variety of herbs and spices to enhance flavor of foods and reduce the need to add salt.
Mixed Berries
FORTIFIED CEREAL
BEANS
Nut Butter
Fluids
Drink plenty of fluids. Fluids can come from water, tea, coffee, soups, and fruits and vegetables.
Grains
Whole grain and fortified foods are good sources of fiber and B vitamins.
Dairy
Fat-free and low-fat milk, cheeses and yogurts provide protein, calcium and other important nutrients.
Protein
Protein rich foods provide many important nutrients. Choose a variety including nuts, beans, fish, lean meat and poultry.
Remember to Stay Active!
Tufts
HNRCA
AARP Foundation

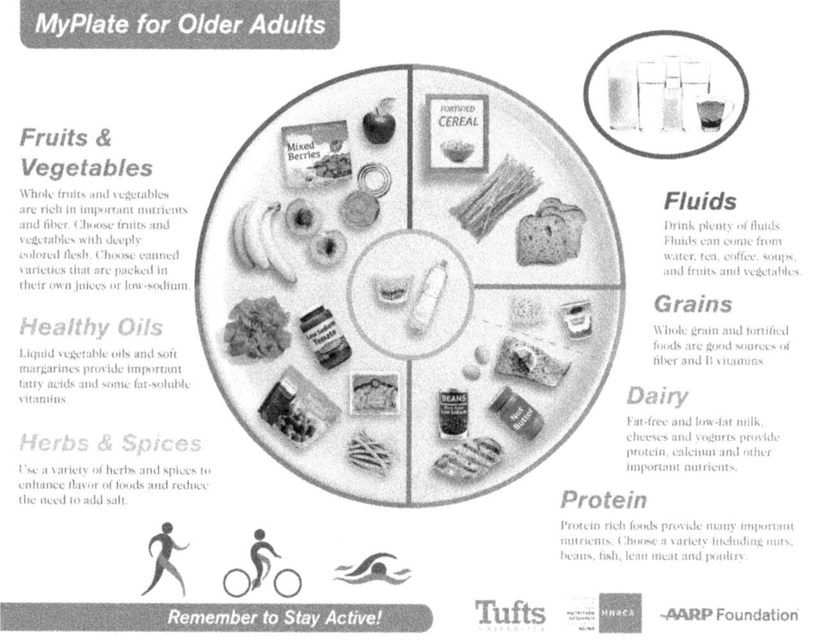

Here are the highlights of a healthy plate from MyPlate for Older Adults:

- Fruits and veggies dominate. Fruits and vegetables fill nearly half of the retooled MyPlate. Dark, leafy vegetables are particularly rich in nutrients, according to panelist Alice Lichtenstein, the vice chair of the 2015 Dietary Guidelines Advisory Committee. Also, plant-based foods are an important source of fiber.

- Colorful choices are healthy. Whole fruits and vegetables with deeply colored flesh are best. Berries, which may protect aging brains, are part of the MyPlate picture.

- Frozen and canned foods are fine. For seniors, canned and frozen foods can be convenient alternatives. They last longer than fresh produce and may simplify portion control. Choose canned goods packed in their own juices or in low-sodium varieties, MyPlate recommends. "Frozen vegetables have equivalent nutrient quality to fresh, but you can get them in bags and just snip them open and pour them out," Lichtenstein said. "So, you can minimize waste, which is important to older adults."

- Calories matter. "As people get older, their need for energy from food—which means calories—decreases," said Lichtenstein. So, strategic food choices include getting more nutrition from fewer calories.

- Salt is off the table. Diners at the congressional event looked for saltshakers in vain. That was a deliberate omission, of course. "As we grow older, our taste buds change," said panelist Lisa Marsh Ryerson, president of the AARP Foundation. "But salt is problematic to our diet and is linked to chronic disease."

- Herbs and spices boost flavor. Who needs salt? A wide variety of herbs enhance the flavor of foods without bumping up blood pressure, panelists pointed out.

- Healthy oils for healthy fat. Liquid vegetables oils and soft margarine fill the center MyPlate circle. That's because they provide an important source of fatty acids and some fat-soluble vitamins.

- Don't forget fluids. Water, tea, coffee, soups and even fruits and vegetables provide essential fluid. "There can be a disconnect between thirst and hydration," Lichtenstein said. "When we're younger, we pretty much get thirsty when we need fluid. When we get older, that's not always the case."

- Protein comes in many sources. Nuts, beans, fish, lean meat, and eggs all provide protein. MyPlate recommends choosing a variety of sources, including certain dairy products.

- Dairy has a place. Milk, cheeses, and yogurts contain calcium, protein, and other nutrients. The key is choosing fat-free or low-fat versions, according to MyPlate.

- Grains give fiber. Whole grains, such as pasta and bread, and fortified foods, including cereal, provide dietary fiber and B vitamins. "For older adults, there's more emphasis on grains—especially whole grains," Lichtenstein says.

- To emphasize the importance of regular exercise for seniors, physical activity is incorporated in the "placemat" section of the new MyPlate with symbols of walking, biking, and swimming.

ChooseMyPlate.gov

MyPlate is a reminder to find your healthy eating style and build on it throughout your lifetime. Everything you eat and drink matters. The right mix can help you be healthier now and in the future. This means:

- Focus on variety, amount, and nutrition.
- Choose foods and beverages with less saturated fat, sodium, and added sugars.
- Start with small changes to build healthier eating styles.
- Support healthy eating for everyone.

Eating healthy is a journey shaped by many factors, including our stage of life, situations, preferences, access to food, culture, traditions, and the personal decisions we make over time. All your food and beverage choices count. MyPlate offers ideas and tips to help you create a healthier eating style that meets your individual needs and improves your health.

Can you see the difference between this MYPLATE and MYPLATE for OLDER ADULTS?

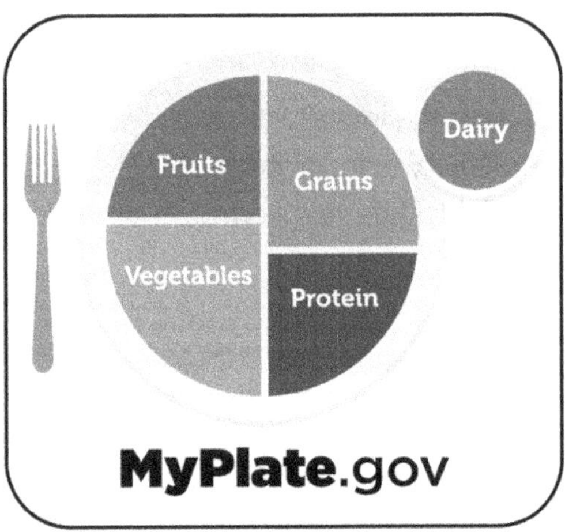

FOOD FOR THOUGHT

Nutrition/nourishment/diet/subsistence/sustenance. These are just words that mean nothing if PLwD are not consuming appropriately healthy nutrients and remaining hydrated. I am providing best practices and not medical or clinical advice; always seek out medical professionals within your circle of care for the unique individual needs of your loved one.

When faced with moving your loved one to a supervised community, it is critical to share their preferences (not just the food component, things like whether they're an early riser or prefer baths over showers). Identify any known physical limitations with their teeth, swallowing capabilities, or ability to manipulate utensils and carve out time to observe staff taking action and utilizing the important information you have provided. By sharing these important details, it will assist in eliminating the regression of the great habits and patterns you have already nurtured, fostered, and created when it comes to nutrition and hydration.

This is a lot of work. It is a full-time job on top of your other full-time jobs. Ask for help, utilize the resources available to you, find out what and who they are, and get on it! Social workers, local senior agencies, and don't forget your community religious chapters—whether they are your spiritual dominion or not, they are there to assist people in need. Don't ever give up on your loved one and don't give up on yourself. You can do it.

Chapter 6

One Dish, Two Dish, Red Dish, Blue Dish

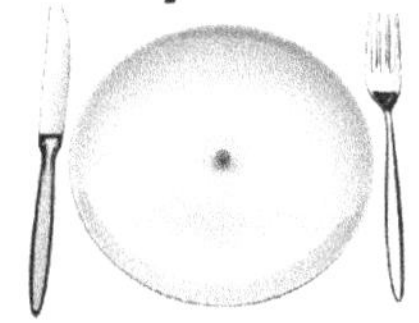

How many components should go on the tabletop or a tray for meal service? What about for People Living with Dementia (PLwD)? Let's see...salad fork, dinner fork, teaspoon, soup spoon, dinner knife, butter knife...NO. If you learn anything from this book, it is LESS is more. PLwD can only process a couple of tasks at a time, so why add clutter to the space?

The planning and consumption of a healthy, nutritious diet are fundamental to a person's wellbeing at any stage of life in addition to combatting other life-threatening diseases as well. Remembering this mantra of "less is more" will assist how you approach and work with PLwD. This chapter provides options on the varieties of service ware and drinking vessels that will ease and aid in the consumption of daily nutrients.

Who's Coming to Dinner?

The Demographic Name Game

The Greatest Generation or Traditionalists are the parents of the "Baby Boomers" and are the children of the "Lost Generation" (those who grew up or came of age during World War I). They preceded what is known as the "Silent Generation," a cohort born between the mid-1920s to the early-to-mid-1940s. The grandchildren of the Greatest Generation are members of Generation X, Generation Y, and their great-grandchildren tend to be Millennials and Gen Z. Confused yet?

The Greatest Generation was a term coined by Tom Brokaw as a tribute to Americans who lived through the Great Depression and then fought in WWII. He said, "That these men and women fought not for fame or recognition, but because it was the right thing to do." Anyone born before 1946 is part of this generation.

Baby Boomers are a designated group of people who were born between 1946 and 1964. They are labeled as Baby Boomers because, during this post-World War II period, there was a statistically significant increase in the number of births that occurred.

Generation X (or Gen X for short) is the demographic cohort following the Baby Boomers and preceding the millennials. The generation is generally defined as people born from 1965 to 1980. As children in the 1970s and 1980s, a time of shifting societal values, Gen X-ers were sometimes called the "Latchkey Generation" due to reduced adult supervision compared to previous generations.

As care partners, these demographics are a reflection of who we are taking care of now and in the near future. Three different generations of age, values, experiences and cultural origins. Before you can effectively care for and manage the activities of daily life of PLwD, you must know who they are as an individual. They are a person who had a family, career, hobbies and well, a fully engaged and functioning life before they arrived at this stage of their life. Never forget the person inside is still there, it is up to us to coax them out so they can shine.

The chart on the next page shows some characteristics of each demographic. Keep this in mind as you work with PLwD, as these beliefs and behaviors are at their core and drive their actions and responses to stimuli. Once you have looked over the chart and made comparisons, the next time you engage with an elder, what would you do/how would you act differently?

Cultural Considerations

If the care partner who is providing feeding assistance has different cultural expectations from those of the person living with dementia, it may reduce the quality of the dining experience (for both of you) as well as their food intake.

For example, in the Korean culture, older adults both expect and are expected to become dependent as a part of normal aging. Such cultural expectations may affect not only the expression and identification of feeding difficulties but also the strategies care partners use to address them. A Korean care partner may provide feeding assistance to an older family member even when it isn't needed because the culture fosters the idea that an adult child feeding a parent is simply healthy reciprocity. By contrast, in Western culture, where greater emphasis is placed on independence, care partners may be more likely to help aging adults to feed themselves. This is

Generational Differences			
	Traditionalist	**Baby Boomers**	**Generation X**
Birth Years	1900-1945	1946-1964	1965-1980
Famous People	Bob Dole, Elizabeth Taylor	Bill Clinton, Meryl Streep	Barak Obama, Jennifer Lopez
Other Names	Silent, The Forgotten Generation	"Me" Generation	Gen X, Xers, Post Boomers, 13th Generation
Influencers	WWII, Korean War, Great Depression, New Deal, Rise on Corporations, Space Age Raised by parents that just survived the Great Depression. Experienced hard times while growing up which were followed by times of prosperity.	Civil Rights, Vietnam War, Sexual Revolution, Cold War/Russia, Space Travel Highest divorce rate and 2nd marriages in history. Post War Babies who grew up to be radicals of the 70's and yuppies of the 80's. "The American Dream" was promised to them as children and they pursue it. As a result they are seen as being greedy, materialistic and ambitious.	Watergate, Energy Crisis, Dual Income families and single parents, Corp. Downsizing, First Generation of Latchkey Kids, Y2K, Activism, End of Cold War, Mom's work, Increase divorce rate. Their perceptions are shaped by growing up having to take care of themselves early and watching their politicians lie and their parents get laid off. Came of age when USA was losing its status as the most powerful and prosperous nation in the world. The first generation that will NOT do as well financially as their parents did.

	Traditionalist	**Baby Boomers**	**Generation X**
Birth Years	1900-1945	1946-1964	1965-1980
Work Assets	Bring value to the workplace with their experience, knowledge. Use their institutional experience and intuitive wisdom to face changes in the workplace. • Consistent • Disciplined • Dependable • Detail Oriented • Hardworking • Loyalty • Stable • Thorough	Politically Savvy-gifted in political correctness. • Anxious to please • Challenges the status quo • Can creatively break down the big picture into assignments. • Good at seeing the big picture • Good team players • Mission oriented • Service oriented • Will go the extra mile • Works hard	Don't mind direction but resent intrusive supervision. • Adapt well to change • Direct communicators • Eager to Learn, Very Determined • Good task managers • Good short term problem skills • Highly educated • Multitaskers • Not intimidated by authority • Thrive on flexibility • Technologically savvy • Value "information" • Want feedback
Work Liabilities	Typically take a top-down approach modeled by the military chain of command. • Don't adapt well to change • Don't deal well w/ ambiguity • Hierarchical • Avoid Conflict • Right or wrong	Challenge Authority of Traditionalists. • Expect everyone to be workaholics • Dislike conflict • Don't like change • Judgmental if disagree • Not good with finances • Peer loyalty • "Process before results" • Self-centered	Don't understand the Optimism of Boomers. • Cynical; skeptical • Dislike Authority • Dislike rigid work requirements • Impatient • Lack people skills • No long term outlook • Respect Competance • Mistrusts Institutions • Rejects rules

a perfect time to reflect on PLwD's life story and ethnic upbringing. What did they witness when it came to their family caring for aging family members? How is this affecting their reciprocity of how they are being cared for now? Are their expectations being met in a positive or negative way? Think about it.

Culture also influences food preferences and mealtime habits. Familiar presentations of foods common to PLwD's culture have been found to improve intake. For example, Hispanic adults with dementia, improved their meal intake when served culturally familiar foods and condiments such as flour tortillas, beans, shredded cabbage, cheese, tomato salsa, and cilantro during meals. It might also help to provide culture-specific eating utensils. PLwD's food preferences may be found in their medical record, but medical records seldom contain information about their mealtime habits, such as whether they prefer to eat alone or while watching television. The most reliable sources for this information are family members and home care partners.

Consider your own family's traditions and "norms" during mealtime. These habits are ingrained in our memory and can be focused on and leveraged to elevate the dining experience to encourage food consumption and promote joyful memories. Don't dismiss the simple things that can make your loved one feel valued, useful, and part of the family dynamic, such as the following:

- Setting the table (establish handwashing prior to the task, the setting doesn't have to be perfect, keep it social)

- Pouring the beverages or water (lightweight pitchers and glasses)

- Tossing a salad and portioning into bowls (keep it simple—do a sample bowl to follow)
- Helping to clear the table (social, social, social)
- Washing the dishes (you can rewash them later if needed)

Promoting Independent Dining

Now we sort of know who is coming to dinner. The more you know about your loved one, the simpler life will be for all. If you know Betty doesn't like green peas, don't serve them—ever. Or if she never wants ice in any of her beverages except her morning milk, well then make it happen every day, especially on your "days off." Take the time to write out a reference list that indicates their preferences, do's and don'ts, and a schedule for snacks and meals—hey, you can't be there 24/7.

The point is that everyone, even those with dementia, has preferences. They also have different physical capabilities. Feeding difficulties are particularly challenging because they can be caused by so many factors, including the following:

- Stiff joints and loss of dexterity due to arthritis can interfere with utensil use.
- Poor coordination and tremors from conditions such as Parkinson's disease can make lifting food or drink or opening containers impossible tasks.
- Limb weakness after a stroke can create challenges with cutting and scooping food onto a fork.

- Visual deterioration caused by conditions such as glaucoma can significantly impact a person's ability to locate food on his or her plate.

- Cognitive impairments or dementia can impact a person's awareness, problem-solving, and motor skills—all making eating an overwhelming task.

Regardless of the underlying cause, self-feeding issues require thoughtful intervention to provide the best opportunity for improved quality of life.

Tool Time

Assistive dining aids can help improve self-feeding ability and promote safety and independence for improving nutritional intake. There are many vendors that offer a wide variety of assistive dining aids for use in feeding programs and to promote feeding independence.

A comprehensive treatment plan should consider PLwD's nutritional challenges and self-feeding ability. Based on these factors, the plan should encourage the least restrictive diet, appropriate positioning, an optimal environment, and any adaptive equipment needed to promote feeding independence.

For your reference, a list and description of assorted types and designs of adaptive eating tools are listed below. Work with your speech therapist and registered dietitian to assist in determining what the best tool(s) to use are and guidelines to follow.

Drinking Cups

Nosey Cups have a cut out for the nose to allow drinking without bending the neck or tilting the head. The Nosey top can also be removed when not needed or during washing.

Two Handle Nosey Cups have a cut out for the nose to allow drinking without bending the neck or tilting the head. The Two Handle Nosey Cup allows for easier holding and manipulation.

The Kennedy Cup is perfect when sitting or reclining in a chair. An easy-to-grip handle can be picked up by those with a weak grasp. The lid screws on tightly to prevent spills or leaks.

The Dysphagia Cup is designed to help prevent liquids from escaping at the lips and directs the liquid to the center of the mouth. Drinking while tucking the chin toward the chest gives normal swallowing mechanisms time to work.

The Two-Handled Cup for Thick Liquids effectively controls the flow of thickened liquid coming from a drinking cup, which is essential for those with dysphagia or head and neck movement concerns. It tips up easily to get the liquid at the bottom without straining or tilting the head and neck.

Convalescent Feeding Cup permits dribble-free drinking without the need to sit up or raise the head. Placing a finger over the vent hole in the cap controls the flow of liquid through the mouthpiece. The design reduces the amount of spilled liquid should a mishap occur. The hole in the mouthpiece is large enough for a straw.

Weighted Two Handle Mug features two large handles that are easy to grasp and a weighted base that helps steady it in the hands of individuals with Parkinson's or other issues that restrict hand control or cause hand tremors. The lid included with the mug has a spout to help control liquid flow while the clear plastic allows for easy monitoring of how much has been consumed.

Utensils

The Plastic-Coated Utensil has a special coating that protects teeth and lips during use. Excellent for PLwD with spasticity or limited hand control.

Coated Bent Built-Up Handle Utensils are all-in-one adaptive special needs dining utensils. There is a lightweight, open-ended steel cylinder design that makes it easier to assist self-feeders. The shaft can be bent to a right or left angle to fit individual needs. The handles are coated with tough plastic for improved grip.

Weighted Utensils feature vinyl handles and a non-skid star-shaped grip that has been designed for comfort. Heavy weighted utensils help stabilize the trembling hand of people with Parkinson's disease.

The ADL Universal Cuff helps enhance the abilities of individuals with limited grip or dexterity control. The cuff has a utensil pocket to hold a variety of items, including eating utensils and writing tools, and straps securely and comfortably on the hand using a soft elastic band for a perfect fit every time.

Soft Built-Up Handle Utensils feature removable foam pads to improve the grip on the utensils.

Comfort Grip Angled Utensils reduce wrist stress. Designed for people with limited upper extremity motion, these utensils feature handles designed for hands with limited grasping ability. They are lightweight, soft, and contoured, and will not irritate pressure points

Finger Loop Utensils are designed for people with arthritis and little or no grip strength. The user places a finger, or thumb, through the loop and stabilizes the utensil with the web of the hand. This configuration allows the hand to be placed in a natural position and provides greater leverage and support.

Plates & Bowls

Round Scoop Dish has a low front and high back to prevent food spillage and help maintain a clean eating environment. Ideal for those with the use of only one hand or other limits to their motor coordination.

The Scooper Plate has a flat bottom and high rim with a reverse curve on one side to help scoop food onto a utensil without spilling over the side. Optional with a suction cup or non-skid base that keeps the plate in place during meals.

The Scooper Bowl features an elevated rim and reverse curve on one side that aids the user in scooping food onto a utensil without spilling. The bottom of the dish has a rubber suction base to provide stability and prevent skidding.

High-Sided Dish makes independent eating easier, especially for those with poor hand coordination, weakness, or tremors. There are two versions: a regular version that maintains the same height all the way around the dish and a cutout edge version that has a sloping side for easier entry of utensils.

Partitioned Scoop Dishes keep food separated and provide more surfaces for scooping. This dish is ideal for individuals who have the use of only one hand or have limited flexibility due to issues with motor coordination, neurological disorders, or ataxia.

Inner-Lip Plates are designed to assist people with limited muscle control and individuals with the use of only one hand. The deep inner lip keeps food from sliding off the plate. The user brings the fork or spoon to the edge of the plate and pushes the food onto the utensil.

Food Guards stop meals from sliding off your plate, fitting snuggly on the plate rim.

This list of tools was actually interesting to put together—who knew? Consider yourself educated on the variety of tools to assist your loved one to independently feed and nourish themself while they still can.

Out of Sight, Out of Sight

In a study done at Boston University over 16 years ago, biopsychologist Alice Cronin-Golomb and her research partners undertook a research study they called, "The Red Plate Study." The idea was to see if seniors with Alzheimer's would eat more from a red plate than a white plate. It has been estimated that 40 percent of individuals with severe Alzheimer's lose an unhealthy amount of weight. It used to be thought that depression, inability to concentrate on more than one food at a time, and an inability to eat unassisted led to this drastic weight loss but in this study, they wanted to see if it could be related to something as relatively simple as being unable to see the food.

While it is known that memory problems are associated with Alzheimer's disease, many people don't realize that vision problems are also an issue among people with Alzheimer's and Parkinson's. Alice Cronin-Golomb said, "If the information getting into their brain through their eyes is already degraded, how can you expect them to do much with that?"

The research team tested people with advanced Alzheimer's level of food intake using the standard white plates and bright red plates. What they found was amazing and significant—PLwD eating from the red plates ate 25 percent more food than those eating from white plates! This relatively simple study has produced hands-on results that family members and care centers can easily implement. As one researcher put it:

"A woman came up to me and said that just the week before, her mother had been in the kitchen trying to pour milk into a mug. The mug was white, the milk was white, and the countertop was white. She poured milk all over the place, and it wasn't until the daughter heard me talk that it clicked in her mind and she understood her mother's vision problem. It's a great feeling to be able to give some information to someone that can make a difference. It's not huge; we are not solving Alzheimer's, but we are helping people in their daily lives."

Following is another article that allows you to understand and embrace what a person with dementia is experiencing.

'Roja Bien!'

"Mrs. A looked at the new red plates and her face lit up. 'Roja Bien!' she commented happily and smiled. After she ate her lunch, she cleaned off her plate, put the utensils on top and stayed at the table, enjoying a cup of tea and conversation with other PLwD."

Makaria Psiliteli, MA, MT-BC, LCAT and Devorah Levin, MPH, RD, CDM, conducted this study on the effects of colored plates in memory care dining. Through the generosity of a grant from New York State Senator Jeffrey Klein's office, they decided to adapt the Red Plate Study for their community. "Since we are a kosher organization and use different plates for meat and dairy meals, we selected the use of red plates for meat meals and blue plates for dairy meals with contrasting placemats. Our interdisciplinary team, led by a clinical dietitian and a music therapist, conducted our informal survey using both red and blue plates in one of our memory care neighborhoods. We used a rated scale as well as qualitative data to determine the impact of the initiative of using colored plates as compared to white plates. We looked at many psychosocial factors, as well as meal intake and PLwD's weight.

Amongst the many positive responses, we found that 60% of PLwD showed an improvement in meal intake while 87% presented with brightened effect and increased socialization during meals. We posit that, in addition to visual contrast benefits, the blue and red dishes helped create a more person-centered, home-like environment for our PLwD. Their comments were positive: 'Pretty plates,' 'Beautiful,' and 'I love the color.' We also observed the excitement of the positive aesthetic change amongst nursing and dining staff."

Final Notes on the Topic of Colors

There is a lot of cumulative data and research across the internet on colors and styles of dishware and drinkware to use. The information shows that there is a significant improvement on the consumption of food and beverage when colors are used. Let me summarize this into four points:

1. Colored plates/glassware allow the food item to "pop" and become visible to the eater.

2. White plates/glassware also work fine if the food is not white or beige.

3. Tablecloths, if used, should be of contrasting color to the plate.

4. Specialty adaptive equipment provides tools for independent eating.

FOOD FOR THOUGHT

The Boston University Red Plate Study and its findings are highly revered. I recommend you work with your speech therapist and listen to their recommendations, particularly regarding the use of adaptive utensils for eating and drinking. Meanwhile, do your own research, and participate in determining the best product and options for your person living with dementia.

My message to you is simple: learn as much as you can about your person living with dementia. Their history, their culture, and for as long as you can, give them the gift of being independent and remaining a participating member of your social group, whether that is your family circle or the community where they are residing. That is the best gift you can provide because sooner than later, that ability to be independent will vanish. #dinewithdiginity

Chapter 7

Swing and a Miss

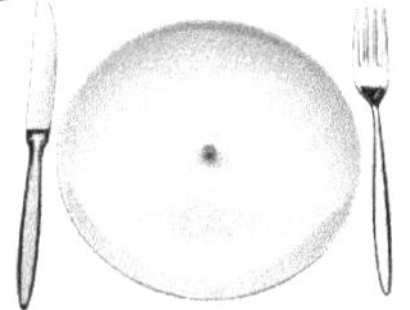

You are likely reading this book because you either directly care for or know a person living with dementia. Have you ever had a bad day interacting with them? No matter what you did, the person's cooperation was at zero, emotions were flying high, your patience was pushed to the max repeatedly, and maybe, just maybe, you might have lost your temper?

If you are having a flashback, breathe slowly and count to ten... The information in this chapter will get your wheels turning on how to not go down that road of emotional pain again—for both the person living with dementia and yourself.

You can't put together a puzzle without seeing the picture as a whole. Sure, we can do the corners first and then the frame, but the other hundreds of pieces look like an overwhelming mountain of guesswork—but in the case of working with PLwD, you can't just toss it back in the box and walk away. It is critical we understand the "why" as we approach the "how" of successfully interacting with PLwD. I want to address your manner and method of personal and up-close interaction via daily care duties and behaviors. Let me clarify when I say behaviors; I am specifically speaking about **yours** and not theirs.

Being a certified trainer of Positive Approach to Care® (PAC™), I have been trained on the techniques and learned they come out front and center in a successful approach to connect and communicate with PLwD. These skills assist and cue not only for the consumption of food and beverage but will also lend to daily care and engagement with PLwD. Let's get started with exciting and eye-opening information for you to ponder and expand your frame of thought as it relates to the action of eating.

Agenda [uh-jen-duh]
Definition: noun, formally a plural of agendum, but usually used as a singular with plural a·gen·das or a·gen·da:

1. a list, plan, outline, or the like, of things to be done, matters to be acted or voted upon, etc.

2. timetable, calendar, program, plan, schedule, diary, lineup, docket, card

We all have busy schedules and responsibilities. Staying organized generally requires an agenda. There is a hardcore, firmly entrenched behavior that all of us have ingrained in our worker bee psyche:

- Start on time/finish on time
- Meet or beat the designated timeframes
- Check off (by hook or crook) that extensive to-do assignment list before your "shift" ends
- Follow the status quo, stay in your lane, do as you are instructed
- Be pleasant, smile, speak in soothing tones, laugh and be a sociable community ambassador

Umm, this pattern of management does not necessarily work when assisting PLwD. When you force your agenda (see above) you will frustrate and trigger a negative response from PLwD. In turn, your frustrations will come out in your voice, body language and with or without a mask—your facial expressions. Now knowing this reality check, reconsider if you have ever said, "I don't know why they hit/yelled/cried/scratch/spit at me."

Training is needed. Lots. Repetitively. In addition to the book, Science of Dementia, there is the cultural and social aspect of taking care of those in need. When Mom starts yelling, you can't wave the medical book at her and expect that will bring her emotions back down from ten to zero. You have to understand what YOU do drives what happens next when you engage with PLwD. You have to make Positive Personal Connections (PPC) and engage the Hand-under-Hand® (HuH™) techniques to redirect.

I will speak of how successful these are in working with PLwD and in deescalating an event later in the chapter. The bottom line is to put PLwD's wants and needs in front of your "agenda." Note: if this is a big cultural shift at home, then have a family meeting and share this paradigm change. Get your core group of family members and helpers involved in this training so the environment can universally relax. Until there is a cure, there is care.

RETROGENESIS: A SIMPLE THEORY

I want to give you another perspective of where YOUR brain needs to go when engaging with PLwD. I'm sure that you have heard the following in one form or another, but please read on. Lightbulbs will go off in your head and this will only help as we dive deeper into getting our folks to eat and drink.

Let me be clear as I share these examples, your person living with dementia is not a child and should not be treated as one! They are grown persons with personal histories and accomplishments that are to be respected. The analogy represents relatable examples of unmet needs when one cannot communicate or express their needs effectively.

Once a man, twice a child - meaning that we start out in life as a child, grow into an adult, then as we age and lose abilities, both physical and cognitive, we become a child again.

So, this was a question asked to a new group of care partners (after learning that the majority have children), "When you brought your brand-new baby home from the hospital and that baby was upset and crying, what do you think was wrong and what did you do to soothe it?" Here are some of their answers:

*Tried to feed them.

*Checked for fever.

*Are they too hot?

*Are they too cold?

*Is the clothing they are wearing too tight? Too itchy?

*Are they bored or lonely?

*Are they constipated?

*They must have their days and nights mixed up, I'm going to try to keep them awake during the day and put them to bed at a certain time each night.

*We've tried everything else; they are still crying. I'm taking them to the doctor.

The baby cries because it has no other way to communicate. When we hear our babies cry, we tend to its needs because we know that there is probably a good reason it is crying. Once we understand our baby's needs, we may become proactive and get the baby into a feeding, sleeping, diaper changing, bathing, or playtime routine.

When someone has an Alzheimer's diagnosis or another form of dementia, they slowly lose the ability to communicate needs as they once did and lose the ability to satisfy their own needs.

We as care partners must learn to identify their needs and either adapt to their routine or slowly get them into a safe and healthy routine. When a baby cries, it probably has unmet needs. When a person with dementia becomes anxious, agitated, sad, or exhibits unusual behavior—it is likely that they have an unmet need and have no other way to express it.

Here are some things you can do to become proactive in meeting your loved one's needs:

Routine, Routine, Routine

1. Establish regular meal and snack times—this is especially important if they also have diabetes to maintain normal blood sugar levels and if they are taking medications for any reason.

2. Establish a toilet routine—incontinence isn't always a result of not knowing they have to use the bathroom. When it comes to someone with a dementia diagnosis, they may not know where the bathroom is, and can't get to it quickly enough.

If we take them to the bathroom every two to three hours or learn their routine/toilet habits, then we may be able to prevent accidents and the anxiety they likely feel when they do know they have to go but have no idea how to get there.

3. Is someone refusing to bathe? What did they do most of their lives—bath or shower? If you are trying to shower someone who traditionally took a bath, you may be fighting a losing battle, so you need to adapt by keeping water out of their face.

Try to accommodate their preference and take into consideration what time of day they typically took a bath or shower.

4. Give them their medications at the time of day the prescription indicates. If you think a certain medication is making them too sleepy during the day, ask the doctor if the time of day can be changed.

Ask the doctor if the medication can be given with food. Some Alzheimer's medications cause stomachaches but are tolerated better when given with food. Some medications cannot be absorbed well if they have just eaten, so find out what the proper time of day is, and if it is best or bad to take with food.

5. Have they had a sudden change in behavior? More confused, agitated, combative, or anxious than usual? Maybe there is another health issue going on, like a urinary tract infection that doesn't always present with noticeable symptoms that a younger person may experience. If the change is sudden and uncharacteristic, get them to the doctor ASAP.

6. Are they asking for someone that isn't here? Asking for their husband, mother, or sister who has passed? Maybe they just need the love that person would have given them at this moment—give them a hug. If they become distressed, follow the training recommendations for redirecting or contact me with any questions, I am here to assist.

7. Have they had a lot of visitors today? Have you taken them out of their routine? Have they had a lot of doctor appointments today? Maybe they have been over-stimulated. Keep visitors to a minimum or set a time limit.

When you have them back in their comfort zone, give them relaxing things to do. Maybe a nap isn't a bad thing.

8. As we age, our body changes and as we become less active, there may be weight gain. Alternatively, if dementia has caused patients to not recognize when they are hungry, they may lose weight.

Our mouths also change over time and dentures may not fit properly, causing problems with eating. Medications and other health concerns may cause edema (swelling) so clothing and shoes feel uncomfortable.

Take them to the dentist and podiatrist, keep track of weight gain or loss, and take those things into consideration when dressing them. Maybe it's time for new clothing or shoes.

As we age, our skin thins and becomes more sensitive—maybe that wool sweater they've worn for years is now itchy. Loose-fitting, comfortable clothing will not only feel better for them but make it easier getting them to change for bedtime or getting them dressed for the day.

Take into consideration that because their skin has thinned, there is less muscle to keep them warm and they may need warmer clothing than you.

9. Troubles with sleeping during the day? Up at night? Set a scheduled wake time and bedtime. Give them things to do during the day, keep them engaged in what you are doing. If you get off schedule for some reason, ease them back into the schedule gradually—this may take up to seven days or more. Changing scheduled medications to a different time of day may help—check with their doctor before doing so.

You've tried everything and still, they aren't sleeping, are anxious, or agitated—make a doctor's appointment, ask for lab work to be done, keep a journal of changes in behavior, sleep patterns, eating habits and share the changes with the doctor.

10. Maybe you need a little extra help. Enlist other team/family members to do the grocery shopping, help prepare meals, take your loved one to appointments, or clean the house so that you can get some relief.

This list of proactive steps is extensive and yes, covers a lot of bases, not just dining. Remember that if they are upset, they won't want to eat/drink and then bing, bang, boom this leads to "situations." The common resolute action is to put on your detective hat to figure out what is driving the swinging behavior.

Remember their brains are shrinking and cognitive health is declining. Some event or thing did happen or change for our loved ones that affected them, and Captain Obvious isn't telling us! Check-in with others in the household or environment of any subtle changes that took place—don't underestimate the impact. A new person or pet in the household, a loud banging door or fire alarm startled and scared them, chairs and tables moved around creating confusion...seems like no big deal to us but we're not the ones dealing with brain change.

Mealtime

We have already discussed different aspects of mealtimes such as the setting, dinnerware, and other basics. Food and beverage consumption will increase when interacting with other people at the table. Social skills will remain with PLwD and be front and center when the opportunity allows.

However, difficulty initiating feeding or aiding during mealtime may take the form of food refusal, aversion to food, or violent reactions to feeding. With food refusal or aversion, they may push the assistance or food away, turn away, spit out the food, or refuse to open their mouth.

Feeding strategies include offering verbal encouragement or sitting down and making eye contact with PLwD. It is wise to either ask them directly or ask family members about their food preferences so that familiar favorites may be incorporated into the diet, or, if those fail, postponing the meal and asking another person for assistance.

On the other hand, if the PLwD's reaction is violent-striking out at you, throwing food or verbally abusing you—the better approach is to put on that detective hat and investigate what may be creating this situation. Are they in pain? Is there too much noise/distractions in the room? Are they frightened by how they were approached (from the side or behind where they can't see you coming while you strap some plastic bib around their necks—think about it)? Rewind what happened before the outburst and what can be done differently going forward.

Time to Eat

"Know thy Person Living with Dementia." "Mom likes lunch in her room. Dad comes in after the news at noon. Mom just laid down for a nap, we will let her rest."

For those PLwD who have habitual patterns and stand waiting in the hallway or sit down early at the dining table, more power to them and you. Don't get agitated because you're not ready (agenda) or it's too soon—give them a cup of tea (hydration) and keep it moving! Ask them to set the table, so what if it's not done "right" or to your standards—dump your agenda! Have unfolded cloth napkins out and ask them to help you by folding them. Engage, engage, engage.

Some PLwD will, however, need prompting; use what we call a Positive Action Starter (PAS). Greet and engage properly, speak slowly, giving them an opportunity to process your statement or question. For example:

- Keep it short and simple: It's time for lunch, Mom. Let's go to the dining room.
- Offer options: It's time for lunch, Dad. Shall I wait, or will you go ahead by yourself?
- Share/help me: Hi Mom, (get their attention), it's Toni. It's noon (you slowly and purposely point at the wall clock or

your watch, they follow your hand pointing). I'm hungry (rub your belly for visual cue), will you walk me to the dining room?

Wait for it, you just had them process:

- Name recognition–theirs
- Your recognition–face/voice/uniform/name badge
- Time of day–try to have a clock with AM/PM visible
- The universal sign of "I'm hungry"–belly rub
- Request for them to help and escort you or self-start to the dining room

The three engagement examples and their actions are taken from Positive Approach to Care® (PAC™), which is where my training and certifications come from. These Positive Action Starters (PAS) connect directly to the Positive Personal Connection (PPC), which in turn may involve the Hand-under-Hand® (HuH™). Lots of alphabet soup but effective, and anyone can master these skills with time and training. I absolutely recommend connecting with me to discuss opportunities for further, detailed training at: https://dinnerWEARhc.info

Daily Activity

Very quickly, here is another option to assisting PLwD in keeping a schedule for themselves, which may include mealtime, medication times, etc. This provides a sense of purpose and accomplishment. Do not overthink this, remember thy person living with dementia and what works for them based on aspects such as their past work history regiments and social lifestyles.

Most options:
Have a weekly calendar posted—use a whiteboard and two different color markers. Fill in the tasks and then go over the scheduled events. Haircut, laundry, garden work, doctor appointments, family member visits... It should not be jam-packed and overwhelming to look at, let alone accomplish. As you learn more about what the person loves to do and how they want to spend their time, the schedule will help fill their day with purpose.

Fewer options:
As the options get fewer, the assumption is the memory and reasoning capacity is decreasing. Have a daily sheet to view versus a whole week, think along the lines of those countdown tear-off calendars. Chances are the tasks will be repetitive such as a bath/shower every Monday/Wednesday/Saturday, daughter visits every Sunday at 1:00 pm. Definitely include at least one item a day to form a habit of looking at the daily personal calendar for structure. Part of the daily task is to hang up the next day's list—engage!

Simplest option:
Provide a general, loosely structured schedule and use the PAS to engage them in choices. Do not underestimate PLwD, the essence of the individual is still in the body; they need your best effort to communicate with them.

Communication: Who's on First, What's on Second, I Don't Know's on Third...

Ever get into a conversation that seems to go nowhere? Bear with me on this, most Boomers will have seen and had a laugh and enjoyed one of the funniest skits on miscommunication ever performed. It is a skit between two people who are talking about the same thing, but when one person has a different perspective, things can get crazy really quickly.

For edification of those who are not familiar with this comedy routine, I will digress for a moment. "Who's on First?" is a comedy routine made famous by the American comedy duo Abbott and Costello. The premise of the sketch from the 1930s is that Abbott is identifying the players on a baseball team for Costello, but their names and nicknames can be interpreted as non-responsive answers to Costello's questions. I think you know where I'm going with this.

For example, the first baseman is named "Who" thus the utterance, "Who's on first" is ambiguous between the question ("Which person is the first baseman?") and the answer ("The name of the first baseman is 'Who'").

Okay, you either know what I'm talking about or I have thoroughly confused you! Google and watch the video for the full effect. This leads me to my takeaway points for communicating effectively:

1. Repeating the question/directions over and over doesn't always work. Try another tact.

2. Raising your voice and physically demonstrating your frustrations will only get you an identical response.

3. Slow it down. Regarding dementia, you can't force someone to remember a person, place, or time. "Yes Mom, you remember Sally don't you? Yes, you do, come on, she was your best friend. You guys used to bowl every Saturday in Brooklyn. What's wrong with you, why don't you remember? You know who I'm talking about." Who is the winner in this escalating conversation? Nobody—you will both feel lousy when it's finally over. Be humble—yield the topic.

Mealtime Assistance

For many people, eating is associated with family, friends, conversation, celebrating, caring, religious events and cultural traditions. Most PLwD face at least one difficulty while eating related to swallowing, seating, eating assistance and amount of food eaten.

We talked about dysphagia previously, but let's expand on understanding what swallowing actually is. Swallowing is the process of moving food and liquids from the mouth to the stomach. We take it for granted because we do it so often and tend not to think about it. However, swallowing is a complicated process.

A Swallow Consists of Three Phases: Oral, Pharyngeal, Esophageal

1. The oral phase. First, food is chewed. Then, the tongue mixes it with saliva into a ball. This food mass is known as the bolus. The lips close to form a barrier so that food can't spill out from the mouth. The back of the tongue and the soft palate form a barrier, preventing food from slipping into the throat before the swallow. The tongue then moves the food to the back of the mouth. During the swallow, the soft palate moves up to shut off the nasal passages, preventing the bolus from ending up in the nose.

2. The pharyngeal phase. The swallow reflex is triggered when the food reaches the back of the throat. Food goes down the throat through the pharynx. The pharynx squeezes to move food down the throat. The Adam's apple will move up and down. Once a swallow is triggered, the epiglottis moves to cover the entrance to the larynx, diverting the bolus away from the airway and towards the esophagus.

3. The esophageal phase. Food enters the esophagus and goes into the stomach.

Did you realize all the steps that unconsciously take place when we eat or drink? The brain change that occurs with dementia interferes with our wiring and our automatic body functions begin deteriorating and losing their effectiveness.

Difficulties at Mealtimes

PLwD can experience various difficulties with eating, including:

- Inability to open food containers
- Inability to see the items on the tray
- Inability to hold utensils
- Inability to cut food or use condiments
- Inability to get food to the mouth
- Inability to organize the meal or complete eating
- Poor or slow chewing
- Inability to maintain a good position necessary to eat properly
- Loss of appetite with less motivation to feed self
- Feeling discomfort while eating
- Impaired swallowing ability (dysphagia)
- Poor concentration on tasks

These problems arise due to various conditions, including:

- Weakness
- Paralysis
- Tremors
- Poor vision
- Lack of coordination
- Memory problems
- Confusion

- Fatigue
- Loneliness
- Depression
- Illness

Major Consequences of Eating and Swallowing Problems:

Malnutrition

This can lead to:

- Confusion
- Poor resistance to infection
- Less responsiveness to rehabilitation therapies
- Skin breakdown and/or impaired wound healing
- Less vitality, a decreased sense of well-being

Dehydration

This can lead to:

- Confusion
- Constipation
- Bladder infection
- Dry mouth
- Severe illness

Aspiration

Aspiration happens when food or liquid passes into the airway, which may cause:

- Chest congestion
- Pneumonia

Airway obstruction

- Choking occurs when food blocks the windpipe so the person is unable to breathe

Non-oral feeding

- Some PLwD will be fed through a feeding tube; this is an individual decision

Description of Feeding Strategies

How and where PLwD take a meal can impact the amount of food and drink they consume. Proper and consistent use of appropriate feeding strategies makes swallowing as safe as possible and minimizes the risk of choking/aspirating. Always get proper hands-on training from a qualified specialist when assisting those who are physically compromised to prevent choking or other serious health hazards.

The following information includes basic strategies to help understand the general steps in feeding physically compromised PLwD.

1. Location

Setting up a good environment lays the foundation for a safe and meaningful mealtime experience.

- Some PLwD prefer to eat in the dining room or their room. Be flexible to their preferences, but be sure to have the ability to monitor their safe food consumption if they are dining solo.

- Reduce distractions in the environment. For some PLwD, community dining rooms are noisy, confusing places.

Decreasing conversations between staff or visitors and turning the radio and television off can help create a calm environment.

2. Sensory needs

These strategies should be used to help PLwD fully enjoy and appreciate meal times.

- Ensure glasses/dentures/hearing aids are worn. PLwD need all of their senses to fully enjoy the taste, smell and look of a meal.

- Get PLwD up just before the meal. This strategy helps PLwD who tire easily, can only sit comfortably for a short period of time, or become agitated while sitting.

- Provide stimulation before the meal. Make sure they are awake and alert before starting the meal. This can be done by stating their name, informing them about the time of day or identifying the foods on the meal tray.

- Use of warm, essential oil-infused towels for their hands or face can be stimulating and signal a meal is on its way. This is a fantastic engagement practice, do it before and after a meal! Always use therapeutic grade essential oils for skin contact or diffusion.

3. Positioning

Proper positioning of PLwD is essential during meals. These are the general guidelines for proper positioning in a chair or wheelchair. Get the appropriate hands-on training from your professional resources such as a physical therapist or whoever your physician recommends.

- Upright and centered.

- Not leaning excessively to one side.

- Pelvis or buttocks should touch the back of the chair to prevent slipping forward.

- Back should touch the chair's back to prevent slipping forward.

- Back should be straight or slightly forward.

- Seatbelt should be secured.

- Feet should be resting on the wheelchair's footrests.

- Inactive arms should be supported on the wheelchair tray or a pillow.

- Head should be positioned so that it is upright or flexed very slightly forward.

- PLwD who are lying back, or who have an arched or hyper-extended neck should not be fed as this creates an open airway, making it easier to choke.

The following general guidelines assure proper positioning in bed while eating. Always get the proper training from a professional to prevent any choking or other serious harmful events:

- Roll the head of the bed up to a 90-degree angle.

- Ensure their body is aligned with and supported by the surface of the bed.

- If they cannot tolerate sitting at this angle, try to position the head at a 75-to-90-degree angle using a small pillow, foam wedges or rolled blankets behind the shoulders, and/or head.

- The head should be positioned so that it is upright or flexed very slightly forward.

Why is Positioning Important?
Positioning PLwD's hips at a 75-to-90-degree angle and the chin tucked downward slightly allows gravity to keep the food bolus (a soft, roundish mass or lump, especially of chewed food) toward the front of the oral cavity. It is important to prevent the bolus from sliding directly to the back of the oral cavity, where it can descend prematurely and increase the risk of choking/aspirating.

Always get proper hands-on training from a qualified specialist when assisting those who are physically compromised to prevent choking or other serious health hazards.

The following information includes basic strategies to help understand the general steps in feeding physically compromised PLwD

- PLwD should never be physically moved by those who have not been trained to do so properly. If they are not in the proper position to begin his/her meal (e.g. turned on one side, moved downwards in the bed), a nurse or trained professional should always be called to help with repositioning.

- Once properly positioned, seat yourself beside and slightly in front of them, so that good eye contact is established. This enables them to maintain the slight chin-tuck position necessary for safe eating. It also promotes social interaction and comfort. Please make sure that they do not tilt the head backward as this opens the airway and places them at higher risk of choking/aspirating.

How Should PLwD be Positioned Once the Meal is Complete?

- After a meal, position PLwD to remain comfortably upright for at least one hour.

- If the person living with dementia is in bed, the head of the bed may be lowered slightly to no lower than a 60-degree angle.

- This helps gravity to promote the downward progress of the meal and prevents reflux of food content that can cause aspiration pneumonia.

4. Set up

There are many considerations when setting up the meal setting area or tray for PLwD. Each of the strategies listed below may help PLwD experience more success when eating.

Always get proper hands-on training from a qualified specialist when assisting those who are physically compromised to prevent choking or other serious health hazards. Food consistencies that have been recommended or ordered must be followed, such as pureed, thickened, chopped, or minced.

The following information is basic strategies to help understand the steps in setting up the meal for consumption:

- Place the food tray in their visual field. PLwD may be unable to see all of the items on the tray if it is not placed where they can see it. At times, it is necessary to place the tray either to the right or left side of PLwD to ensure all parts are visible.

- Place the tray within reach. To encourage independence and participation during the meal, place the tray within PLwD's reach. Always place the food and utensils on their stronger side.

- Cut food into appropriate sizes. PLwD may be unable to use a fork and knife, so need you to cut food into bite-sized pieces. Be sure to follow the physician's order regarding the ordered mechanical consistencies of food and drink. *Cut the food in the kitchen before serving to keep it at the proper serving temperature.*

- Lids and containers should be opened. Making a meal accessible increases the likelihood of all items being eaten. Opened juice and milk containers will increase PLwD's chance of receiving appropriate fluid intake. *Remember if your hands are coming into contact with food (e.g., opening wrapped bread to butter it) be sure to put on a fresh pair of gloves to prevent cross-contact or cross-contamination!*

- Put soup in a cup. This strategy increases independence for PLwD who can pick up a cup but are unable to use a spoon to carry a thin liquid. *Be wary food temperatures are not too hot to prevent burns. Ensure the proper cup is used (handles) and the contents, if physician ordered, are pureed to prevent choking.*

- Provide straws. Straws increase independence for PLwD who cannot hold a cup but can easily reach a straw. Please check with the doctor's orders first, as some PLwD with swallowing problems may not be allowed to use a straw for drinking.

- Remove unnecessary items from the table setting or tray. This strategy helps PLwD focus on the important items that need to be eaten. For example, remove lids and wrappers, and leave only the utensils and food.

- Give only one item at a time. Position one dish at a time in front of PLwD to reduce confusion or impulsivity. We always want to encourage independent eating.

- Provide adapted utensils. When appropriate, ensure special utensils are available at every meal and are washed and sanitized after every meal.

5. Nutrition and hydration

Nutrition and hydration strategies can be used during meals where food intake is less than usual due to illness, fatigue, or other factors.

Always get proper hands-on training from a qualified specialist when assisting those who are physically compromised to prevent choking or other serious health hazards.

The following information is basic strategies to help understand the general steps in feeding physically compromised PLwD:

- Consult your physician or registered dietitian for guidance on the best meal planning for your loved one.

- Give high-calorie items first. Items on the menu/tray are fed in high- to low-calorie order to ensure the most valuable intake occurs. Feed entrée first and when they have had enough, provide nutrient-dense fluids (e.g., supplements, fortified pudding, and milk). Follow with soup, tea, coffee, or any combination of these items.

- Arrange for small, frequent snacks. Snacks may be required for PLwD who eat slowly or become tired easily. Focus on protein-based snacks, not sugary and salty junk food.

- Provide water for PLwD with swallowing difficulties. PLwD may complain of thirst after receiving thickened fluids or tube feedings. Even with hydration requirements met, they may continue to experience the sensation of thirst and/or dry mouth. Before serving water to PLwD on thick liquids, please check with your physician, nurse or speech-language pathologist to make sure it is safe to do so.

6. Verbal encouragements and directions

There are many ways to help PLwD eat. Our loved ones may simply need help understanding what is on the table/meal tray, what to eat next and how to eat it. Verbal prompts are important and can help guide them through all the steps of a meal. At times, PLwD may only require encouragement or praise for trying.

- Identify foods on the tray by name or taste. This helps PLwD who have difficulty seeing the plate/tray and its contents. Best to remove multiple choices and focus on one food item at a time.

- Help PLwD get started by telling them where the food is or which utensils to use. Best to remove excessive items for clarity.

- Prompt them on what to do next. PLwD who have trouble knowing the next step to eating will need you to tell them what to do. Get their attention by addressing them by name and mimic the next action step to get started. Be patient.

- State the person's name as often as necessary. PLwD who are easily distracted or tend to drift off during the meal may benefit from having their names called to alert and redirect them to the task of eating.

- Praise and encourage PLwD. Everyone likes to know they are doing well. Encourage PLwD to continue what they are doing right. Encourage please and thank you's!

7. Physical guidance

Some PLwD may only be able to participate in feeding at certain times, or can only complete certain aspects of feeding. Independence during mealtimes should be encouraged whenever possible. Don't forget their field of vision shrinks as the disease progresses. They may not even see the item you are encouraging them to consume. Here are some ways you can provide physical guidance to PLwD:

- Be sure you have their attention and place the food on the spoon and hand it to them. Some PLwD are able to move their hand to their mouth for eating but cannot get the food onto the utensils properly. By placing the food on the spoon and then handing it over, you are encouraging person to play an active role in eating.

- Hand the cup to them. PLwD who cannot get started may need you to hand them a cup in order to drink. They may not be able to reach for the cup on their own but are able to hold it and drink from it. Be aware of the temperature of hot items to ensure they are tolerable.

- To encourage participation, hand finger foods to PLwD. For some, it is not always obvious that finger foods, such as a sandwich, can be picked up. *Use gloves!*

- Initiate and then allow them to take over. Help PLwD get started, as they may only need help to begin eating rather than be fed the whole meal. Keep an eye on them to ensure they are chewing and swallowing before adding more food to their mouths.

- Take turns. Take turns with PLwD in getting food to the mouth. Alternating gives them the opportunity to participate, learn from your actions, and receive additional support. Mealtime assistants should establish and maintain a controlled rate of intake during the meal.

- Provide Hand-under-Hand® (HuH™) assistance helps guide PLwD. This technique also helps to maintain attention and level of alertness. Get educated by a certified independent trainer to maximize your effectiveness at https://dinnerWEARhc.info.

8. Spoon-feeding

PLwD who require complete spoon-feeding need to be observed carefully during feeding. When providing spoon-feeding, it's important to consider PLwD's perspective to ensure the proper bolus size and rate of feeding. Consider the use of a "coated" metal spoon which has a special plastic coating to protect lips, teeth, and gums.

Always get proper hands-on training from a qualified specialist when assisting those who are physically compromised to prevent choking or other serious health hazards.

The following information is basic strategies to help understand the general steps in feeding physically compromised PLwD:

- Provide teaspoon-sized bites and sips. A metal teaspoon is usually the best utensil for spoon-feeding because it provides the appropriate amount of food. PLwD should be provided with one teaspoon-sized bite at a time and fully swallow the bite before having another.

- Slow the rate of feeding. Slowing the rate of feeding gives PLwD more time to prepare the food in the mouth and to swallow. If food is introduced too quickly, the muscle sequence for swallowing can be disrupted, leading to aspiration. PLwD who require spoon-feeding often have difficulty swallowing and require additional time to fully clear the bolus from the mouth and throat.

- Allow time for two swallows between mouthfuls. Most people swallow more than once per mouthful. Watching or feeling for the up and down movement of the Adam's apple can help identify when they have swallowed.

- An empty mouth does not always mean that food has been swallowed; the food may simply be out of sight at the back of the tongue or pocketed in the cheeks. Providing extra time allows for extra swallows to occur, as each may take a few seconds or longer.

- Recognize requests for more and indications that they have had enough. PLwD set the pace of the meal by indicating readiness for more food and drink. Completed swallows, a nod, a verbal request, or an open mouth are all indications they wish to continue eating. Whenever possible, offer PLwD a choice of what to eat next. If they appear to be getting tired, are nodding off, or are swallowing slower, break from or stop feeding until they are alert enough and ready to continue.

- Gently rub the spoon on their lower lip. Rubbing the spoon gently on the lower lip may encourage mouth opening. Try to allow PLwD to remove the food from the spoon with their lips; this encourages participation.

- Feed the unaffected side of the mouth. PLwD's muscles may be weakened on one side of the mouth (e.g., due to a stroke). These PLwD should be fed to their preferred side to take advantage of stronger, more coordinated mouth muscles that help with chewing.

- Alternate taste, texture and temperature of food. Varying these characteristics may assist in increasing awareness of food in the mouth, particularly for PLwD who have trouble remembering that food has been placed in the mouth.

Consistent Mouth Care After Meals

At the end of each meal, please ensure that the mouth is empty and no food is being pocketed (e.g. in the cheeks or under the tongue).

Monitoring For Signs of Eating Problems

It is important to always watch for signs of eating problems. Any of the following observations may indicate swallowing problems and should be reported to your loved one's physician/nurse or speech therapist:

- Coughing/choking during meals
- Frequent throat clearing during eating or drinking
- Wet or gurgly voice during meals
- Excessive drooling
- Vomiting
- Nasal regurgitation (food or drink coming from the nose)
- Complaints of pain when swallowing
- Chest congestion around meals
- Holding lips tight
- Food spilling excessively out of the mouth
- Holding food in the mouth
- Refusing to eat

Refusal to eat should not be interpreted as uncooperative behavior. Mealtime assistants are not to force–feed PLwD. Please report the refusal to eat to the physician/nursing staff so that the appropriate assessments and referrals can be completed.

Choking- Emergency Procedures

Get certified in basic CPR and the appropriate first aid, encourage and include all family members to get certified also. Always get proper hands-on training from a qualified specialist when assisting those who are physically compromised to prevent choking or other serious health hazards.

Stop feeding immediately and seek immediate medical attention or call 911 if PLwD experiences these conditions:

- Excessive coughing
- Gagging/gasping for air/struggling to breathe
- Grabbing at the throat
- Turning blue in the lips and face
- Indicates that something is stuck in his/her throat

In all cases of choking, stay with PLwD at all times and follow this procedure:

- STOP feeding
- Shout for help, seek immediate medical attention or call 911 depending on your location
- Keep them in an upright position
- Do not pat them on the back as this action could push the food further down into the airway

Follow your established household or community emergency response protocol. If you successfully address and resolve the choking situation, you should still immediately report and notify your physician/nurse for any next steps.

Mealtime Strategies

Goals and roles of the mealtime assistant (either yourself or a professional caregiver):

1. Provide nourishment, understand their capabilities, needs and diet restrictions.
2. Help PLwD be as independent as possible and maintain his/her dignity.
3. Be an active participant in PLwD's eating experience by creating a social event every time.
4. Learn PLwD's mealtime style, be flexible and patient.

5. Have a helpful attitude, take an interest in them—smile, engage in light conversation, describe the meal. Make eye contact and use the skills you have been taught to assist them.
6. Take time to feed or assist PLwD to eat a well-paced meal.
7. Know PLwD's strengths and difficulties, and build on the strengths to compensate for the weaknesses.
8. Teach PLwD new skills to enjoy mealtimes. Coach, assist and encourage independence.
9. Follow the recommendations of the community care team and review PLwD's care plan regularly. Watch for any changes in PLwD's eating pattern and report them to your professional care team for assessment.
10. Ask the care team for advice if you are having trouble following the recommended feeding strategies. They are a resource for you, please establish a relationship and communicate on a regular basis.

Who plays a role in facilitating safe feeding? If your loved one is in a care community, the round-the-clock staff are there to serve and care for them. Everyone has a role in supporting each other as the care plan is developed and modified as needed. You are not on an island; seek direction from your physician or seek resources from a social worker.

The following are some of the common support team positions with a short description of their skillset:

Certified Dietary Manager, Certified Food Protection Professional (CDM, CFPP)

CDM and CFPPs are experts at managing food service operations and ensuring food safety. They are responsible for applying nutrition principles, documentation of nutrition information, implementation of menus, food purchasing and preparation.

Speech-language pathologist (SLP)
Speech-language pathologists provide a primary role in a clinical swallowing evaluation to recommend appropriate diet texture and feeding strategies.

Communicative disorders assistant (CDA)
With proper training and supervision from a speech-language pathologist, communicative disorders assistants help feed PLwD.

Registered dietitian (RD)
Registered dietitians provide individualized nutritional care to PLwD. Nutrient intake and appropriate food choices are determined with the recommended food and drink consistencies in mind.

Occupational therapist (OT)
Occupational therapists address seating and positioning needs and prescribe adaptive eating devices.

Physical therapist (PT)
Physical therapists consult about posture, trunk/upper extremity strength and range of motion related to PLwD's ability to self-feed.

Physician (MD)
Physicians are responsible for overall medical management and educating the care team and families about the effects of certain diseases on swallowing and eating. Physicians regularly review medications and medical treatments to determine if these affect eating and swallowing.

Registered nurse (RN) and registered practical nurse (RPN)

Registered nurses and registered practical nurses identify appropriate PLwD for the Mealtime Assistance Program and notify the care team and volunteers when there is a change in PLwD's swallowing status. Nurses supervise and support mealtime assistance given by family members, private caregivers, and volunteers, and suggest improvements to eating strategies.

Social worker

Social workers communicate eating concerns to PLwD, family, and the healthcare team.

Recreation therapist

Recreation therapists oversee recreation programs where food may be served.

Pharmacist

Pharmacists assess the potential impact of medications on swallowing and eating and assist the registered nurse and speech-language pathologist to assess medication administration.

Note: please do not confuse any of this information provided with training on how to be a certified and paid feeding assistant—it is NOT.

FOOD FOR THOUGHT

The word "agenda" should have a different meaning for you by now. Take the steps needed to move it to the back of the bus. This chapter has been important in the explanation and highlighting of actions you may not have considered before. As care partners, we must be made aware of the numerous choices and service options we can control as we strengthen our understanding of how PLwD can be positively impacted.

As a PAC Certified Independent Trainer, I make several references to the Positive Approach to Care® programs and techniques in this chapter as well as the book in general. I firmly believe that by educating yourself and those around you with these methods, it will improve your loved one's quality of life, along with yours. If you would like more information, please visit my website https://www.dinnerwearhc.info.

Chapter 8

What's on the Menu?

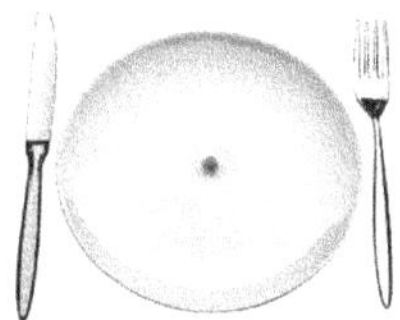

Menu Recommendations

Each stage of dementia can usher in new challenges for those living with dementia and their care partners, especially in dealing with one of the most critical daily activities—nutrition. We have covered several areas regarding nutrition, dysphagia, environment, and service ware. It's time to get down to the actual food and food safety.

Food Safety and Good Hygiene

Food should be stored, prepared, and presented in a safe and hygienic environment. Extra care is needed for people who are ill or have weak immune systems as they may have a lower resistance to food poisoning.

Everyone should properly wash their hands with soap and water before and after preparing food, especially raw proteins and other potentially hazardous foods. Your hands should be washed before you help people to eat, touch silverware, glasses, or china, when removing the soiled dishes and cleaning the surrounding dining area such as the table, chairs, etc. Gloves serve a purpose but create their own form of chaos and danger if not properly worn, changed, or disposed of.

This is a good opportunity to utilize the warm hand towel infused with essential oils for your loved one. They will enjoy the warmth of the towel and enticing scents while cleaning their hands on their own. It would be a nice start (and finish) to the meal when you both sit down and do this ritual together (watch what I do).

10 Quick Tips on Keeping Food Safe

ServSafe.com and FoodSafety.gov are excellent and easy to navigate websites for all food safety information. Have your entire circle of care partners review and understand these basic rules of food safety...the life you save may be your own.

1. Wash hands with soap and water

Wet both hands with clean running water and apply soap. Use warm water if it is available. Rub hands together to make a lather and scrub all parts of the hand for 20 seconds. Rinse hands thoroughly and dry using a clean paper towel. If possible, use a paper towel to turn off the faucet.

2. Clean, wash, rinse, and sanitize surfaces

Clean: Remove debris.

Wash: Surfaces should be washed with hot, soapy water.

Rinse: Use a clean towel and water to remove the soap/cleaning chemical

Sanitize/Disinfect: Use the EPA list to determine if your sanitizer/disinfectant solution meets and exceeds the COVID-19 requirements. Apply and allow sanitizer to air dry unless noted otherwise. ALWAYS follow the usage directions for any chemical and have the Safety Data Sheets (SDS) readily available for first aid and disposal/spill information.

3. Clean your refrigerator daily

All products (technically speaking) should be dated upon delivery with month/date/year (when shopping/receiving your purchases or deliveries, always check the manufacturer's expiration dates). Products should be stored on a first in first out (FIFO) basis. Any time you break the seal on a package, it must be wrapped, labeled, and dated. When in doubt about the quality of the product, throw it out.

4. Rinse produce

Rinse fresh vegetables and fruits under running water just before eating, cutting, or cooking. Even if you plan to peel or cut the produce before eating, it is important to thoroughly rinse it first to prevent microbes from transferring from the outside to the inside of the produce.

5. Separate foods when storing in refrigerators or freezers

Place raw seafood, meat, and poultry in plastic bags, sheet pans or sealable containers. Clearly label the use-by date so FIFO can be followed—reducing spoilage and waste. Follow the standard of the order in which to store proteins, always keeping ready-to-eat (RTE) foods above raw protein-based products. This should be followed in the freezer as well. If the unit breaks down and the product thaws, blood will not drip onto RTE products, which will then have to be discarded.

6. Separate foods when preparing and serving

Always use the designated, clean cutting boards for fresh produce and proteins. For home use, try to have a red or colored board for raw food and a whiteboard for RTE (ready to eat) items. Have enough cutting boards on hand and replace those that are scarred and have cracks in them as they harbor bacteria which leads to food-borne illnesses. Avoid cross-contact and cross-contamination.

7. Use a food thermometer when cooking and holding food for service

A food thermometer should be used to ensure that food is safely cooked, and that cooked food is held at safe temperatures until eaten. Thermometers should be calibrated daily with an approved cleaning/sterilizing process in place for food thermometers.

8. Cook food to safe internal temperatures

One effective way to prevent illness is to check the internal COOKED temperature of seafood, meat, poultry, and egg dishes before serving. Guidelines are available on the aforementioned websites and should be readily available for reference. Remember, PLwD probably already have compromised immune systems and undercooked proteins will make them sick. And by sick I mean potentially vomiting and diarrhea, which will be misery for everyone.

9. Keep foods at safe temperatures

The temperature danger zone is 41°F to 135°F. Keep hot foods hot and cold foods cold. Hold cold foods under 41°F and keep hot foods at 135°F and above. Invest in a $5 bi-metal food thermometer—not to be confused with an oven thermometer. Clean and sanitize your thermometer in between temping different food proteins, items, and storage. Do it.

10. Sick people stay out of the kitchen

Friends and family members exhibiting signs of illness must be removed from the kitchen and dining environment immediately. People exhibiting symptoms of vomiting, diarrhea, jaundice (go to the doctor immediately), sore throat with fever and any infected open wounds should be quarantining from everyone until they feel better and exhibit no symptoms for 24 hours. Protect our people with compromised immune systems from getting unnecessarily sick.

Food safety is definitely a bigger topic to review outside of these 10 tips. This is the shortened home version. Care communities are under review of a regulatory agency and have much higher standards and required certifications in order to be compliant to keep PLwD safe.

When in doubt, visit ServSafe.com and FoodSafety.gov for additional information or clarification on food safety questions.

Diet Texture Categories

The texture of food and drinks can be altered to make chewing and/or swallowing easier and safer for our elders. PLwD with swallowing difficulty are assessed by a speech-language pathologist to determine the most appropriate diet texture. The International

Dysphagia Diet Standardization Initiative (IDDSI) has created an international standard of food preparation terminology, along with the implementation of the program, and service standards. The Academy of Nutrition and Dietetics (AND), beginning October 2021, will recognize IDDSI as the only texture-modified diet noted in the Nutrition Care Manual (NCM)®, which is a professional practice resource for registered dietitian nutritionists. Listed below are brief descriptions of the current commonly used diet texture categories, in addition to the IDDSI terminology:

Solids

Regular textures/EASY TO CHEW EC7 or REGULAR RG7

All solid foods, including those that require excessive chewing. For example: sandwiches, roast meats, salads, whole fruits and vegetables.

Soft textures/SOFT & BITE-SIZED SB6

Most solid foods, except those that require excessive chewing. For example: soft-filled sandwiches, soft meats, soft-cooked vegetables and fruits. Be advised on the consumption of bread for those with chewing and swallowing issues (soft, minced and pureed diets). Bread can become gummy and sticky in the throat and hard to swallow, creating an opportunity for choking—check with your speech therapist or registered dietitian for advice.

Minced textures/MINCED & MOIST MM5

Soft foods cut into small pieces. For example: ground meats, pasta, cooked and diced vegetables.

Puree textures/PUREE PU4, EXTREMELY THICK EX4

Mashed foods that require minimal chewing. For example: puréed vegetables and meats, mashed potatoes, and puréed dessert.

Liquidized food/LIQUIDIZED LQ3

Liquidized foods may be used if the PLwD is observed having trouble moving their tongue, giving them more time to "hold and move" the liquidized food as they process the swallow.

Liquids

Thin liquids/THIN TN0

Most regular drinks, including those that move quickly when poured. For example: broth soup, coffee, tea, milk, juice, and water.

Thick liquids/SLIGHTLY THICK ST1 or MILDLY THICK MT2 or MODERATELY THICK MO3 or EXTREMELY THICK EX4

Drinks that have been thickened to a honey or nectar consistency and move slowly when poured. Mildly Thick MT2 is known as Nectar Thick and Moderately Thick MO3 is known as Honey Thick. For more details and information go to www.IDDSI.org. For example: thickened juice, thickened water, and cream soup.

Mixed consistencies

Pieces of solid foods within a thin liquid. For example: vegetable soup, cereal with milk and fruit cocktail.

Planning Meals and Snacks

When thinking about the sorts of meals and snacks that PLwD might eat each day or each week, there are some key things to think about:

- A variety of foods should be served.
- Combinations of colors will make the food attractive. Three or four areas of color look good on a plate.
- A combination of different textures increases the appeal. People who don't have chewing or swallowing problems will appreciate crisp, crunchy, chewy, smooth, and soft foods.
- Tastes should be varied, but meals containing too many different or new flavors may not be acceptable to some people, especially those with dementia, who may appreciate more recognizable or traditional foods.
- Some finger foods, as well as foods that require cutlery, allow variation at mealtimes.
- Always keep in mind any cultural themes that will appeal to your population of PLwD—make it an event to keep the socialization aspect highly engaging.
- Finger foods should not be pigeon-holed as just sandwiches cut in quarters for the memory care segment. Remember when fried or baked macaroni & cheese balls came out? Everyone loved the novelty. Think out of the box when preparing your meals to meet the needs of PLwD.

Beverages and Hydration

What if fluid intake is a problem? The body is about 60% water, give or take. You are constantly losing water from your body, primarily via urine and sweat. To prevent dehydration, you need to drink adequate amounts of water. There are many different opinions on how much water you should be drinking every day.

Health authorities commonly recommend eight 8-ounce glasses, which equals about 2 liters, or half a gallon. This is called the 8×8 rule and is very easy to remember. In general, 8 to 10 cups of fluid (4 pints) should be included every day to keep well hydrated. On hot days, when sitting in centrally heated areas or if there is an infection present, try to encourage an extra 1 to 2 cups.

During the early stages of dementia, a person may simply forget to drink because they are less sensitive to thirst and/or cannot recall when they last took a drink. Those with moderate dementia often have difficulty remembering the mechanics of how to drink, such as turning on the faucet, where the glasses are stored, or even how to get fluid into a glass.

The risk of dehydration is most severe in the advanced stage of dementia due to not recognizing one's thirst, having a complete loss of thirst or being unable to express thirst to others. Consider putting pre-measured multiple bottles/glasses of water in key areas of PLwD. This is a good way to keep track of how much water/liquid is being consumed daily and you can make adjustments as needed.

Signs and Symptoms of Dehydration

Increased confusion and/or a change in usual behavior are the first signs that someone with dementia may be dehydrated. Additional behavioral changes associated with inadequate fluid intake include weakness, fatigue, agitation, muscle cramping in the arms and legs, nausea, and dizziness.

Changes in urination such as infrequent urination and/or dark amber or strong-smelling urine can also signal dehydration. Certain medications and vitamins can make urine darker, so be sure to look at the overall symptoms. It is important to note that dehydration increases the risk of a urinary tract infection, which can cause an acute phase of confusion.

Tips to Stay Hydrated

Be proactive and never assume that someone with dementia will ask for a drink. Leave beverages out in visible areas as a reminder to drink up, always take water when out and about, and find fun and tasty ways to slip liquids into the day's activities. Great choices include:

- Offering small amounts frequently, about half or ¾ a cup at a time if larger amounts are not being taken.
- Using flavored ice-cubes made with juices to add extra flavor and fluids.
- Enhanced water works great; use fruits, herbs, and vegetables to make water more appealing. Lemon or orange slices, cucumber, mint, assorted berries, and assorted

melon can not only add flavor, but if in a display vessel, adds visual appeal. If adding fruit to individual glasses, consider pureeing the fruit (not the herbs) and adding before serving to prevent any choking hazards.

- Placing the cup in the person's hand as a prompt if needed.

- If someone has a familiar or regular cup that they prefer, try to encourage its use.

- Remember fluids include soup, tea, fruit juices, diluted or fizzy drinks and water. A variety can help to maintain interest in drinking. Make it a point to reduce the amount of sugary or "diet" beverages, there are so many flavored seltzers that can be used as replacements.

- Utilize fruits and vegetables with a high-water level content. Leafy greens, celery, berries, melons, cucumbers, tomatoes, and apples are easily incorporated into their diets.

- If you are unable to be there to prompt the person to take fluids, try making up a jug or bottle of juice and placing it within view. Ideally, try to use a clear plastic jug or bottle so that the fluid can be seen.

Most of us think dehydration is a worry for hot summer days. The truth is, dehydration can happen any time of year if you aren't taking in enough fluids. As little as a two percent loss in body fluid that isn't replaced can lead to mild dehydration. The result can be headaches, constipation, problems concentrating, sluggishness, and fatigue.

If a senior you love has Alzheimer's disease or another form of dementia, poor hydration might be a daily struggle they (and you) will have to contend with. It's important to address the issue, and more importantly, stay ahead of it.

Snacks

Care partners can supplement the meals of PLwD by providing nutrient-dense snacks that appeal to the eye, nose, and taste buds.

It is important to remember that some snacks should be tailored to their individual needs if they have a medical condition such as diabetes or trouble chewing, so be aware of any chronic or potential choking and aspiration conditions they may have.

Snacks that are high in salt, sugar, fat or excess calories without nutrition should be avoided. Skip the convenience products also and prepare these from scratch. This allows you to put that extra touch on it which may drive whether they eat it or not. Would you rather be handed a wrapped or lidded container or have a fresh, visually appealing granola bar or fruit yogurt cup?

Here are some examples of nutritious snacks PLwD may like:

- Greek yogurt or cottage cheese—jazz it up in a clear cup and garnish with fruit
- Assorted cheeses and crackers—vary the cuts and types of crackers
- Sandwiches made with deli meat like chicken breast or salads like chicken salad—cut into wedges or fingers, or piped onto mini pita or naan bread

- Granola or breakfast bars, especially the homemade softer varieties; use a high protein recipe
- Fruit or fruit/vegetable juice blend beverages—turn this into a social activity with tastings, get their opinions on flavors and colors
- Nuts or trail mix—be aware of choking hazards or do assorted nut butters
- Vegetables (parboil the veggies if they have trouble chewing raw) and dip—watch the fibrous and stringy veggies like celery or asparagus
- Smoothie or milkshake with fruit/vegetables—interactive bars; get the high quality, low noise blenders so everyone doesn't jump out of their chairs every time you turn it on
- Pudding or gelatin snack cups—make homemade ones and get kooky with the visual and flavor mixes; put inside empty sugar cones so they can hold in their hands and eat
- Fruit cups packed in their own juice—use fresh fruit and puree a complimentary fruit for the juice e.g. strawberries with watermelon juice
- String cheese sticks, cut from cheese blocks so you can make different shapes
- Antipasto kebabs with pretzel sticks (not the wooden skewers), cured meats, cheese, olives

- Raisins, yogurt covered raisins, craisins, dates, or figs; be aware of who you are serving these to as they are choking hazards for some folks
- Fresh fruit: orange and apple wedges, grapes, pitted cherries—make sure the fruit is ripe and sweet-tasting; take the peels off
- Hardboiled eggs or deviled eggs
- Fig or fruit newton style bars—homemade, of course
- Hummus and pita
- Custard or flans; use a high protein recipe
- Ice cream, pudding pops or fruit juice bars—put muffin papers on the ends to catch the drips
- Wheat or fruit mini muffins with freshly brewed coffee
- Glass of chocolate milk or buttermilk served in a special glass
- Avocado on toast

To make life easier for you, focus on the planning. Plan your snacks on a documented rotation schedule. This will help with purchases and preparation. Also review the rotation to compliment that day's menu—meaning if the menu is bread heavy (pancakes, muffins, cornbread, cakes), then have the snack be of a lighter nature. If carrots are on the meal, don't offer carrot sticks and ranch dressing as a snack—make sense? Keep the colors in mind and have a variety of textures to further promote interest—chewy, crispy, cold, hot, etc.

For Your Consideration

Before we dive into the topic of the meal itself, let's discuss other contributing factors to providing nourishment for PLwD.

What if the person is struggling to complete meals?

- Allow extra time for meals as needed. Each individual deserves about 45 minutes.
- Serve one course at a time to keep food temperatures palatable, this also helps to avoid confusion with foods.
- Prompting, such as giving verbal advice or placing cutlery or a cup in the person's hand, can help.
- Prompting also helps to maintain dignity and independence for as long as possible. As the condition progresses, it may be necessary to assist with eating.
- Dish up a small amount of food at any time. Once eaten, a further portion can always be served.
- Consider offering five to six small snacks during the day rather than three main meals.
- Consider plate warmers or insulated cups to keep food and drink warm for longer.

- When people with dementia are eating together as a group during mealtime, avoid removing plates until everyone is finished. Removing plates early can be seen as a signal to stop eating.

What if wandering or becoming easily distracted at meals is a problem?

No matter how hard you try, it can be difficult to get someone to eat a plated meal if they are unable to sit down long enough to complete it. The constant movement from pacing or agitation will also burn up extra energy and can contribute to weight loss. If they like walking, let them walk, but ensure that the snacks they have travel well. Try:

- Leaving out snacks along the route the person walks or place food in their hand to prompt them. Try a variety of finger foods (see the section on finger foods for suggestions). Always remember to follow food safety rules when leaving snacks out.

- Encouraging high-energy food where possible, see the section on adding extra energy and protein.

- Changing the environment. Some people will benefit from the television or radio being switched off to limit distractions.

- If you notice that there are times in the day when the person is more settled, consider changing the times for meals or offering additional snacks at these times.

Adding Extra Energy and Protein

Adding extra energy and protein can be a challenge, especially if the amount someone will eat is small. The answer is not always to add extra foods, instead try changing the way food is offered or using foods such as butter, sugar, full cream milk or jam to add extra energy and protein. You can also try to:

- Avoid low calorie, reduced-fat, or reduced sugar foods unless you have been advised otherwise by your health professional.

- Add extra butter, grated cheese, soft cheese or cream to potatoes, soups, sauces, or vegetables to add extra calories without increasing the volume.

- Spread jam, honey, marmalade, and butter thickly on bread, toast, scones, bagels, croissants, waffles, and pancakes.

- Use whole milk or cream in cereals, sauces, puddings, and drinks aka "Super Cereals."

- Add a teaspoon of jam, syrup or honey to hot cereals, custards, rice pudding or porridges.

- Fortify whole milk or creamers by adding two tablespoons of milk powder and use as normal in cereal, sauces and drinks. This will help to add energy and protein.

Please note: the suggestions regarding adding extra fats and sugars are extreme recommendations. Please check with your registered dietitian for oversight and approval before making any changes to the menu choices.

What if Constipation is a Problem?

It is important to encourage good bowel health as constipation can reduce appetite and contribute to increased confusion and agitation. Food high in fiber helps bulk up stools and make them softer and easier to pass. Try:

- Including extra fruit and vegetables—such as a side salad, diced or pureed vegetables in savory sauces or dishes, stewed fruit, dried fruit or chopped fresh fruit such as a banana with cereal, fruit as a snack or fruit juices with meals.

- Including snacks that contain fiber, such as cereal bars, a handful of dried fruit, multigrain or seeded crackers.

- Using whole wheat/grain bread and cereals.

- Have soups that contain beans, lentils, or peas.

If fiber is being increased, this should be done gradually to avoid discomfort and excess flatulence. At the same time, fluids should also be increased. Aim for at least 8 to 10 cups of fluid per day, which will help make stools easier to pass. Working with your RD contributes to the oversight and monitoring of any changes made in diet orders, consumption, and results.

Now, The Menu

Miniature versions of foods are often better than cutting up larger items, as this creates a more stable product that is less likely to fall apart. Finger foods are generally not expensive: the goal is to use basic ingredients to create smaller, flavorsome, and transportable items.

Using finger foods in place of traditional meals may prolong a person's independence and stimulate them to eat more frequently. These foods can be eaten easily, without the need for cutlery, they hold their form when picked up and require limited chewing. Serving handheld foods for people with moderate to severe dementia is a way to help preserve dignity, increase self-esteem, and enable independence at a time where mobility or coordination may be limited.

When people are eating with their fingers, it is a good idea to encourage hand washing and have wipes available before and after meals to minimize food contamination and gastric upset. Warm towels that are scented with essential oils will set the stage for the meal. It will accomplish the handwashing task while stimulating the senses with the warm towel and essential oil benefits.

Of course, when implementing finger foods as part of a menu, the issue of choking needs to be considered. Remove seeds and skins, ensure soft and moist items are available for those with difficulty chewing or swallowing, and continue to provide adequate mealtime supervision. Avoid toothpicks and other sharp objects such as kebab skewers.

Sample Finger Food Menu

Take your existing menu and get creative with modifying to handheld items. Open your mind, include your entire family as you discuss and create alternative choices. The following is a sample of an all-day menu complete with snacks (for the record this is a broad example of suggestions, I did not calculate the nutritional content for the day):

Breakfast

Cereal bar, 5 dried prunes, 1 glass of orange juice, tea/coffee, OR

Hard-boiled egg (shell removed), 1 to 2 multigrain pieces of toast (cut into strips), 1 glass of milk, 1 banana, tea/coffee

Morning Snack

Orange wedges, tea/coffee, OR

Cheese cubes and savory crackers, tea/coffee

Lunch

Beef sliders with cheese and lettuce in buns with thick-cut chips, ice cream in a cone, water, juice, OR

Mini salmon patties with sweet corn relish, rice balls, green beans, cut-up fresh fruits (remove skins and seeds), water, juice

Afternoon Snack

Mini fruit muffin, tea/coffee, OR

Naan with peanut butter and jam, milkshake or smoothie

Dinner

Thin pureed soup (e.g. chicken and vegetable soup, served in a cup) with bread and butter, fresh zucchini slices or sticks (cooked or raw), served with cherry tomato (halved), carrot/celery sticks, fruit juice, water, OR

Thin pureed soup (e.g. beef and noodle soup, served in a cup) with bread and butter, grilled chicken strips, tortilla wrap and yogurt dip, romaine leaf salad, fruit juice, water

PM Snack

Warm milk drink and cookies or sweet biscuit, OR

Milk drink and toast with butter

Handheld/Finger Food Ideas

I can literally provide hundreds of recipes for you. Look at some of the ideas noted below and you can easily surmise what the original (regular) menu item is. A lot of these items can be served to the entire family for dinner or extra portions can be labeled, dated and frozen for a later meal.

Breakfast

Sausage & Potato Empanada

Ham & Cheesy Egg Bites (muffin tin or mini loaf pan)

Pancakes with Bacon (cooked bacon strips placed in batter before the turn)

Waffles & Sausage (waffle iron used, add cooked sausage crumbles in batter)

Lunch & Dinner

Egg Salad Pinwheel (10" tortilla, cut in half for serving)

Baked or Fried Macaroni & Cheese Balls (add ground ham)

Pork Schnitzel Fingers (ground pork)

Baked Salmon Lettuce Cups

Hot Ham & Swiss (oven bake with slider buns)

Lasagna (muffin tin)

Chicken & Rice Balls (ground chicken aka porcupine balls)

Sides

Pasta & Vegetable Salad (large pasta-ziti/rigatoni seasoned, marinated blanched veg, composed on a plate—easy to pick up a la carte)

Corn & Bean Salad (in toasted bread cup/phyllo dough/puff pastry)

Coleslaw (in toasted bread cup /phyllo dough/puff pastry)

Spinach & Potato Patties (griddle/pan fry)

Rice Balls (plain seasoned rice that is hand-packed shaped)

Polenta Sticks/Wedges

Orzo Balls (deep fry or cheesy baked)

Key Culinary Tips for Handheld Foods Program

The mission of this program is to assist PLwD maintain independence in eating and stabilizing or increasing their nutritional intake while improving overall satisfaction with mealtime. This satisfaction is achieved from the manner in which we assist PLwD during meal or snack times and getting them to actually consume the food, hopefully on their own accord. Utilizing the Positive Approach to Care® and Hand-under-Hand® techniques are essential to making this happen. Contact me for coaching at https://dinnerwearhc.info

Prep & Production

There are no limits to what you can do in creating handheld food. Look over the list below and your mind should start racing with ideas coming together in your head of what you can do. As with all food production, keep food and physical safety needs front and center when holding and serving food.

- Soups are pureed thin and served in mugs for drinking (no chunks or choking hazards and watch the point of service temperatures!)

- Sauces, syrups, gravy can be served on the side for dipping. Be sure the ramekin or dipping dish is a color to allow these items to be easily seen. (e.g. a black ramekin for syrup doesn't work)

- Breakfast bread items can be cut into strips or quarters. Fresh batter items you can add diced, cooked breakfast meats into the cooking process.

- Use a sandwich maker for sealed food pockets of hot or cold items. Change up the bread and the filling. Watch the temperatures for food safety.

- Utilize mini muffins, regular muffins, and mini loaf tins for numerous menu items.

- Premade doughs can be utilized in the tins or by themselves as a vessel to hold fillings.

Hot Soups and Cereals

The hot soups and cereals, if served in mugs, should not exceed your normal hot beverage serving temperature—between 110°F and 130°F. DO NOT confuse cooking and holding temperatures with serving temps. Either break out that food thermometer (that you have been sanitizing in between uses) and check the temperature or just taste test it yourself before serving.

Muffin and Mini Loaf Tins

These are going to become your best friends! There are so many sizes and styles available now, including silicone and different shapes. My biggest word of advice—do not cheap out on these tins and if getting silicone molds, be sure they are food grade. My favorite is a little pigs in a blanket silicone baking mold.

- Breakfast: pancake batter with cooked sausage or bacon crumbles inside

- Lunch/Dinner: corn muffin mix with cooked chopped franks, ham, BBQ chicken

- Snack: cake batter with mini peanut butter cup or use as a jello mold

See what I'm getting at? You can do anything you want, don't hold back. Get your family together and start brainstorming.

Sandwich Makers

These are the coolest multi-function machines to have. Most of them come with different plates so you can do sandwiches, waffles, and a basic griddle. These are perfect for cooked-to-order food for meal, snack, and dessert items. Research the product and manufacturer choices and invest in a quality, heavy-duty piece of equipment—you will be using this tool for all three meals plus snack time!

Suggestions

- Toasted sandwich pockets of any kind. You can put cold filling and press, put hot filling on the bread and press, and check out the recipe book that will come with a maker for ideas.

- Pizzas made with seasoned Italian bread filled with sauce, cheese, meats, and veggies. Serve extra sauce on the side.

- Cinnamon raisin toast filled with cream cheese and jelly or peanut butter for a quick snack.

Can you imagine the wonderful aromas that will be generated? Let's get busy people! Do the research to ensure you get the best sandwich maker for your needs. Develop and test the recipes, train your family members, engage PLwD too. This can be a total social and fun family event to use this tool for fresh, delicious and easy handheld, finger food items.

#diningwithdignity

Is this a lot of work to do to provide food options for PLwD?

In the beginning, yes—but mainly because it is different and breaks from the norm.

In the end, no—practice makes perfect and after all, you may learn a few new things that everyone can enjoy. Be a true partner in care for PLwD.

#diningwithdignity goes further than just the food. Dining is a social event. The symbolism and distraction of the use of the institutional bib, plastic liner or napkin tied to an alligator clip chain around your loved one's neck are appalling. We can do better by our people by using sustainable, reusable cotton DinnerWEAR Dining Scarves. Check out my website at https://dinnerwearhc.info

#diningwithdignity is the practical and thoughtful use of the Positive Approach to Care® techniques that assist, encourage, and enable PLwD to feed themselves, even if it just for a small moment of time. There is still that wonderful and loving person inside, just waiting for an opportunity to shine.

#diningwithdignity is what we do to enrich lives, theirs and our own. Self-value improves when we make the effort to make a mealtime special. Everyday. For everyone.

FOOD FOR THOUGHT

You have been provided with an untapped alternative way to serve food for all PLwD. Engage your loved ones in a manner and setting that normalizes their meal or snack time. Get your entire family and friends involved in recipe development and the actual steps of cooking and tasting.

By the way, eating with your fingers is okay. Embrace it and leave your AGENDA at the door. Change your mindset. Make it special by offering warm hand towels that are infused with therapeutic grade essential oil before and after the meal. Diffuse these therapeutic grade herb, mint, and citrus oils before the meal to engage PLwD with wonderful smells to jump-start appetites and uplift moods. This is an opportunity to elevate your dining experience, not dumb it down. #diningwithdignity

Chapter 9

OMG What About Me?

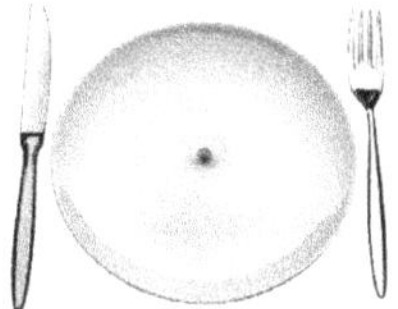

Care Partner Support

You Are Not Alone!

Today, there are an estimated 5.7 million People Living with Dementia (PLwD) in the United States and over 16 million people caring for them. It's a challenge many more of us will face, as either patients or care partners, as the population ages. The diagnosis of dementia is life-changing, both for the people living with it and those who care for them. Dementia is complicated. It can affect all the senses. It can impact memory and comprehension. It can cause anxiety, fear, and often mistrust of other people, including care partners.

Knowing what your loved one (or the person you are caring for) is experiencing at each stage of dementia will help you keep them safe, comfortable, and meaningfully engaged. This guide for dementia care partners was designed to provide you with the knowledge you need to care for PLwD, insights about how it affects you and your loved one, and practical steps you can take to manage your role as a care partner.

What You Need to Know About Being a Care Partner

Your First Priority as a Care Partner

The first person any care partner needs to care for is themselves. When you become a care partner, you assume a responsibility that can be physically, mentally, and emotionally draining. Being a care partner may strain your patience, your finances, and your time. It can lead to a range of feelings that can be, at a minimum, uncomfortable, and in the extreme, unhealthy.

Don't be surprised by your negative feelings about having to care for someone with dementia; it can take you for a ride on an emotional rollercoaster. Even the calmest individuals can experience a range of negative emotions. Hey, you're only human.

You may feel:

- Overwhelmed
- Confused
- Depressed
- Isolated
- Desperate
- Alone
- Trapped

- Guilty
- Angry
- Grief-stricken
- Frustrated

None of these feelings are unusual. The best way to handle them is to acknowledge that they are a natural reaction to a stressful and challenging situation. If they persist, reach out to an Alzheimer's support group in your community, a family physician, clergy, or a therapist for help. Don't neglect your own personal mental and physical health.

10 COMMUNICATION TIPS FOR DEMENTIA CARE PARTNERS

Communication—the expressive or receptive exchange of information—is vital to the functional success and emotional well-being of a person with dementia.

Yet difficulty expressing needs and/or understanding another person is common when someone has Alzheimer's disease or another form of dementia. Communication breakdowns can be extremely stressful for both the person with dementia and the care partner. They can also contribute significantly to excess disability.

But you have the power to communicate effectively with someone who has dementia—throughout every stage of their disease—by adapting your communication style. Never underestimate the powerful impact you have on someone you provide care for. As a care partner, you are the most important tool for facilitating a positive experience for the person and for you.

When it comes to communicating with someone who has dementia, ask yourself: "How can I adapt to this person, instead of them adapting to me?" I will also mention that you will have to check your "agenda" at the door and be flexible when working with PLwD.

Use the tips on the following pages to adapt your communication style, and you'll help improve the person's function, emotional well-being, and quality of life at every stage of their disease.

TIP 1: Gain Attention and Trust

Before you speak, make sure you have gained the person's attention. It's also important that the person in your care feels safe with you and that you have his or her agreement and approval to proceed. They may not remember your name or who you are, don't let this stop you from treating them with respect and love.

Leave your own feelings of rejection and sadness on the curb (agenda). Chances are they may get a memory spark and recall who you are, you can never tell. Blame the disease that is shrinking their brain, and don't take your anger and frustration out on them—be ready for the spark.

EXAMPLES: "Good morning, Mom. It's Betty. It's time to go to breakfast." "Hi Mom, would you like to take a walk or watch TV?" "I'm (your name), and you are...?"

Offer options and make a Positive Personal Connection®.

TIP 2: Approach From the Front/Side

Always try to approach a person with dementia from the front/side so he or she has an opportunity to recognize you. I say front/side so you don't close off their total field of vision, effectively blocking off a perceived "escape route". Keep in mind too that in the later stages of dementia, the person's range of vision may become more limited, so you may need to make further adaptations.

Before speaking, make direct eye contact (unless it's culturally unacceptable) and stand or sit in front of the person so that you're at their eye level. Maintaining eye contact during the conversation helps show that you're listening. It also builds trust, promotes respect, and lets the person know that you care about them.

Remember with the reduced vision, their limited range of vision means they cannot see you coming from behind or swooping in from the side and you will likely startle them. Think binocular or monocular vision capability.

TIP 3: Minimize Distractions

People who live with dementia are often easily distracted by both sights and sounds. Before communicating, try to eliminate all unnecessary sources of stimulation. If you need to handle someone's personal belongings, be sure to ask his or her permission first.

EXAMPLES: "Mom, can I take your sweater to the laundry?" "Hey Dad, can you turn the volume down on your radio?" "Helen, let's put these magazines away until after lunch."

TIP 4: Lead With the Person's Name

Calling a person with dementia by their name shows respect and identifying yourself often helps the person with orientation. Leading with the person's name will also catch their attention, improving their ability to attend to your question or request.

EXAMPLES: "Hi Mom, it's Carrie. Are you ready to play cards?" "Good morning, Ethel. You have a beautiful blouse on today, I love that color." "George, it's Becky. Can you help me fold these towels?"

TIP 5: Avoid Pronouns

Referring to a book as "it" or to a person's son as "he" can seem logical to someone who does not have a cognitive disability. But for someone who has dementia, pronouns can often frustrate and confuse them. What is "it," and who is "he"? To be clear, speak clearly. Use simple sentences, and avoid words like it, he, his, she, her, them, they, those, etc. as much as possible.

EXAMPLES: "Marvin, is Arlene here?" (not "she") "Caroline, can you put your shirt in the basket?" (not "it") "Tony, let's give the books back to Jerry and Allen." (not "them")

TIP 6: Use Short Sentences

Long sentences filled with lots of information can be confusing to someone with dementia. A sentence like, "Turn the water on and wash your face because your daughter is coming to see you this afternoon and we want you to be freshened up before her visit," will most likely not be fully understood. Keep your sentences short and to the point.

EXAMPLES: "Bob, your son Billy will be here soon." "Mr. Gibson, turn on the water please." "Barbara, use the blue towel, thank you."

TIP 7: Wait for a Response

Research shows that response time for a person with dementia can be delayed by up to 30 seconds. For you, as a care partner, this delay might be frustrating sometimes. It's also easy to misinterpret a delay as the person's inability to comprehend your message. Be patient.

Remember to speak slowly and keep questions short and sweet—don't overload their capacity to interpret what you are saying. When communicating with someone who has dementia, allow time for them to process your words. During processing, do not distract the person. Be patient and you will often receive the response you might have otherwise missed.

TIP 8: Use Visual or Tactile Cues

Words alone may not be enough to convey the meaning of your message. This can lead to a lack of response and the conclusion that the person cannot or will not do what you're asking. Use visual demonstrations and tactile/hands-on cues to illustrate your words.

EXAMPLES: While saying, "Please brush your hair," demonstrate the movement of a brush on your own hair. While saying, "Raise your arm," raise your own arm to demonstrate.

TIP 9: Watch Your Nonverbal Messages

A key aspect of communication is nonverbal. In addition to the words you use, your tone of voice, volume, body language, and facial expressions also send a message every time you speak. Nonverbal messages can be both intentional and unintentional, so be careful not to change the meaning of your message with your nonverbal cues.

EXAMPLES: Keep your volume at a normal level (unless the person is hard of hearing). Avoid crossing your arms, as this can indicate impatience or tension. Remember that a smile is often contagious.

TIP 10: Be Patient, Supportive, and Friendly

At every stage of dementia, there is a person behind the patient. When it comes to how someone with dementia communicates, let them know that they have your full attention. Focus on the feelings related to their communication, not just the facts.

Whenever possible and appropriate, use additional forms of communication to express support, such as touches and smiles.

Remember that good communication brings rewards to both the sender and the receiver.

Dementia Care Do's and Don'ts

DO:

- Be the calming constant for the person with dementia to temper their anxiety
- Be present in the moment with your loved one
- Encourage conversation and laughter; it may be slow in coming, but don't give up
- Use your hands when talking to show actions because words may not be enough
- Enjoy music, rhythm, dance, prayers, and poetry together
- Walk along with them when they wander; they may have a need but are unsure how to meet it, e.g. they may want to find their bed, get a drink, or go to the bathroom but cannot verbalize it
- Offer choices but limit them to just two at a time
- Help them get started with a task (because sometimes they forget how to start)
- Find friends, family, and care partners that they like to be around; it takes a team

- Let others take over care sometimes, so you can refuel yourself as the main care partner

- Encourage drinking water and other liquids; dehydration is a problem

- Ensure a safe environment when your loved one is unaware of hazards, e.g. loose rugs, inadequate lighting, electrical sockets

- Ensure your loved one can swallow foods without choking; choking can indicate a need to change food textures to remain safe

- Understand that your loved one is going to continue to change...they are still the same person, but different

- Understand that you cannot grieve for your loved one in front of them; they are anxious and do not understand; be the positive and calm presence in their life

- Learn to say, "I am sorry; this is hard" and de-escalate their anxieties when they get upset; it's kinder and more respectful, so you both can move on

DON'T

- Attempt to reorient your loved one to the present, if they are in another time and place

- Feel guilty when you must stretch the truth to accommodate a potentially stressful or confusing situation

- Mistake dementia for stupidity; your loved one isn't stupid, they are just living with brain change
- Hesitate if it's time to take the keys away; your loved one would take them from you if your positions were reversed
- Feel selfish for taking time for yourself away from your loved one
- Expect your loved one to start following your directions if you weren't someone who gave them directions before; know that you may get your feelings hurt
- Be frustrated when your loved one cannot complete an activity today that they could do yesterday; sometimes each day is different
- Argue over trivial matters; understand what is happening and just let it go
- Change topics too quickly; your loved one is behind in processing what they hear, so they will respond slower and struggle to keep up
- Feel angry when your loved one swears or uses inappropriate words; they are using the abilities they still have
- Ask open-ended questions that require a specific answer–instead of, "What do you want to drink?" say, "Would you like a hot or cold drink?"
- Speak in "baby talk" or high-pitched tones; use a calm, deeper version of your voice to reduce anxiety

- Tell a person living with dementia that someone they are looking for is dead; they will relive the grief each time. Many patients will ask, "Where is my mother?" Instead of saying she has passed, say, "Tell me about your mother" and give them the opportunity to talk about how that person made them feel.

FOOD FOR THOUGHT

Get to know the person's life story and preferences BEFORE it's too late. Family members, please make this a priority while your loved one can still participate and communicate their desires. What do they or don't they like to eat and drink? Likes and dislikes for their daily care and routines? Adapt to their cognitive level—they will still have preferences but cannot engage in those activities independently.

By shelving our agendas (must eat breakfast by 8:00 am, must wear the brown shoes and not the black ones), and adapting to the needs of the person we are caring for, we will arrive at our destinations together in a peaceful fashion. Shift your thinking. Be willing to make mistakes (and forgive yourself), work to change your own brain, be open to possibilities and change!

Let's Get Back to You—Caregiving is Rewarding but Stressful

Six simple strategies and tips to maintain your well-being

The emotional and physical demands involved with caregiving can strain even the most resilient person. That's why it's so important to take advantage of the many resources and tools available to help you provide care for PLwD. Remember, if you don't take care of yourself, you won't be able to care for anyone else.

To Help Care Partners Manage Stress:

1. Accept help. Be prepared with a list of ways that others can help you, and let the helper choose what he or she would like to do. For instance, a friend may offer to take the person you care for on a walk a couple of times a week. Or a friend or family member may be able to run an errand, pick up your groceries or cook for you.

2. Focus on what you can provide. It's normal to feel guilty sometimes, but understand that no one is a "perfect" care partner. Believe that you are doing the best you can and making the best decisions you can at any given time.

3. Set realistic goals. Break large tasks into smaller steps that you can do one at a time. Prioritize, make lists, and establish a daily routine. Begin to say no to requests that are draining, such as hosting holiday meals.

4. Get connected. Find out about caregiving resources in your community. Many communities have classes specifically about the disease your loved one is facing. Caregiving services, such as transportation, meal delivery or housekeeping may be available.

5. Seek social support. Make an effort to stay well-connected with family and friends who can offer nonjudgmental emotional support. Set aside time each week for connecting, even if it's just a walk with a friend.

6. Set personal health goals. For example, set goals to establish a good sleep routine, find time to be physically active on most days of the week, eat a healthy diet and drink plenty of water.

7. Seek professional consulting. Before you lose your temper and lash out at your family. An all too typical scenario: family members who can't or don't want to acknowledge that Mom or Dad struggle with daily life and are declining. They aren't around to see and feel the results of rough times when your loved one is out of sorts and not cooperating. "I just don't see it. What are you talking about? Everything's okay. What's the big deal?" Get professional help for your own peace of mind and sanity because it only gets harder as the disease progresses.

8. Take time off and get away consistently. An hour, half-day, overnighter maybe. Just make time for yourself to recharge and let your hair down without looking over your shoulder. Could be an awesome cup of coffee on the boardwalk at sunset. A funny movie. Go bowling and hurl that ball down the lane with a vengeance (get a kiddie ball so you don't throw your shoulder out). A meal at your favorite restaurant where you leisurely dine and enjoy the food (go easy on the alcohol). Do something for yourself, you sure as heck earned it. Hang in there my friend.

FOOD FOR THOUGHT

This type of care, work and responsibility isn't for everyone. It is emotionally and physically challenging every day. You are special, don't ever forget it. Give yourself a break every once in a while for criminy sake. But, arm yourself with information and take advantage of any training offered to increase and improve your skills and thicken your armor. The disease of dementia will continue to progress and get worse, I promise you. Stay strong, hydrate, eat well, exercise your body and mind, and get plenty of rest to rejuvenate. Speak honestly about how you are feeling and channel your frustrations to people you can trust, lean on and garner support from. Thank you for everything you do! Until there is a cure, there is care.

Afterword

Buckle up Buttercup

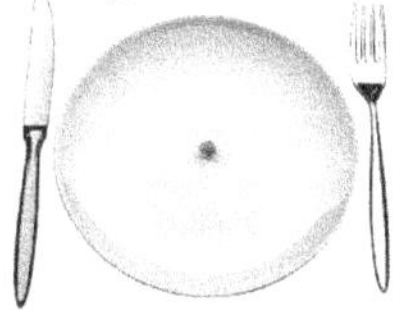

People Living with Dementia (PLwD) are everywhere. They can be a neighbor, a friend, or a family member. There are also different stages and different types of dementia with almost 10 million new cases every year. If you are reading this book, you have taken an important step to maintain and extend the health and wellness of your loved one and yourself. A friend of mine said it best, "If I did it wrong today, I have another chance to figure it out tomorrow." Never give up.

I am unabashedly a food service expert. In my spare time, I studied, trained, and tapped into a lot of excellent, professional resources to ensure I was on the right path when composing this tool. This is not a clinical book. This is an everyday person's guide to approaching dining and dementia. The substance of the book provides education, insight, and recommendations for actionable options. Actions that you can implement immediately.

This is a book you can read and learn from and move the needle on how you manage and care for your loved one living with dementia. Oh, and by the way, your life will get a little bit better too. Take a moment to jot down your biggest challenges and dive back into the book for a recommendation. If you don't see what you need, contact me, I'm here for you.

It is expected an estimated 10 million baby boomers will develop Alzheimer's. Of those who reach the age of 85, nearly one in two will get it. Unless we find a treatment or a cure, Alzheimer's will become the defining disease of the Baby Boom generation. They will be Generation Alzheimer's. Too many of America's Baby Boomers will spend their retirement years either with Alzheimer's or caring for someone who has it.

So, what can you do about it? Get educated, learn how to care for yourself so you can provide care for those who are afflicted with this deadly disease. Become a true care partner. Anticipate and engage. Arm yourself with knowledge of how to navigate this journey of brain change to enrich everyone's life for as long as you can.

FOOD FOR THOUGHT

Now here's the good news. Until there is a cure, there is care. The world (and the business) of dementia care is constantly changing. Learn and embrace what I am providing to use as a guide for new best practices, so you can truly do what is best for that person who is living with dementia.

About the Author

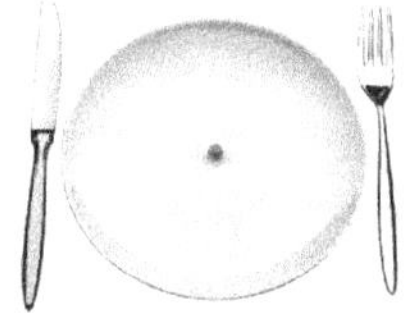

Toni Fisk is an Air Force Brat who grew up outside of Atlanta, Georgia, sowed her wild oats in Orlando, Florida during the '80s and moved to Long Island, New York in the '90s where she met her husband and started her family. Toni has worked in the dining industry her entire career, beginning in hotels as a Server to Restaurant Manager, and later transitioning to the world of Healthcare and the Senior Living sector in various roles ranging from Executive Chef to Operations Vice President.

Working with our elders in skilled nursing communities gave her the raw and unfiltered experience of dementia and how it was being managed, and some of the failings spurred her into action. Every community is different, but there is always the opportunity to raise the bar on care; this is what prompted Toni to get her numerous certifications for dementia education and training. This knowledge and insight combined with her years of being a dining subject matter expert are exactly what is needed to open the eyes and minds of Care Partners nationwide.

Toni continues to pursue her mission of improving the quality of life for all our folks dealing with brain change, as well as those who care for them. She creates fidget quilts and dining scarves to add to the socialization and daily care needs of our elders. Toni has been published in several professional magazines and anticipates more books in the future on topics related to the every-persons journey of caring for our People Living with Dementia.

Toni's credentials include: Positive Approach to Care® Certified Independent Trainer, Second Wind Dreams Virtual Dementia Tour® Certified Trainer, ICCDP Certified Montessori Dementia Care Professional, NCDDP Certified Dementia Practitioner, ANFP Certified Dietary Manager, Certified Food Protection Professional, and NRA ServSafe® Registered Instructor and Exam Proctor, yet it is her passion for grace and kindness that blazes the trail.

You can visit and connect with Toni on her website https://dinnerWEARhc.info for more information on dementia and dining operations training, as well as her other products.

DinnerWEARhc, Inc

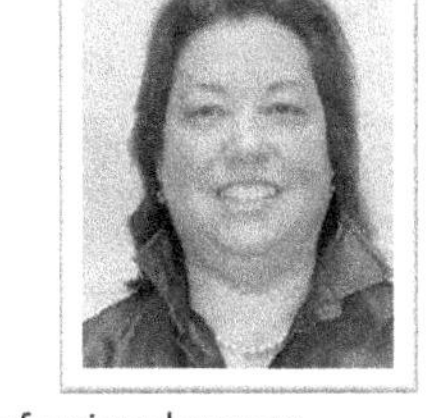

Toni Fisk, Principal

www.linkedin.com/in/tonifisk

Professional Summary

Toni has been engaged in the food & hospitality industry for over 35 years, her professional career encompassing Walt Disney World/EPCOT Center and Marriott Hotels before transitioning to Healthcare and Senior Living. Toni has always embraced the "Servant Leadership" model as she ascended the ranks during her career; whether being a Server or Dining General Manager, Executive Chef or Operations Vice President, Toni has always practiced inclusion, communication and professionalism.

Toni's daily operational engagement at Senior Living Communities across the United States stoked a concern regarding the care, training and tools that were accessible to all the pillars of support services who were caring for our elders, particularly those living with dementia. This was the foundation for DinnerWEARhc, Inc. Initially, the core business was dignity-based clothing protectors and fidget quilts, growing to dining operations quality initiatives and food safety, then going to the next step of dementia education and training for enhanced dining activities. Toni is a published author who provides speaking engagements and training workshops for family caregivers and residential community staff members.

Employment

Principal, DinnerWEARhc, Inc., Consultant • Valley Stream, NY • February 2018 – Present
Vice President Operations, Senior Living, Unidine Corporation • Boston, MA • July 2014 – January 2018
District Manager, Sodexo Senior Living • Simsbury, CT • 1986 – 2014

Education

ICCDP Certified Montessori Dementia Care Professional
NCCDP Certified Dementia Care Practitioner
Teepa Snow Positive Approach to Care® Certified Independent Trainer
Second Wind Dream Virtual Dementia Tour® & DACE® Certified Trainer
Certified Dietary Manager, Certified Food Protection Professional
ServSafe® Certified Instructor & Proctor
Dietary Manager Certification, Adelphi University • NY, NY

Publications

- ***#dinewithdignity Unlocking the Mystery of Dementia & Dining***
  Published book releasing Spring 2021
- ***Why Isn't Mom Eating***
  Positive Approach to Care® Online Journal 2021
- ***Boosting Your Memory Care Dining Experience***
  Association of Nutrition & Foodservice Professionals EDGE Magazine March 2021
- ***Dining and People Living with Dementia***
  Association of Nutrition & Foodservice Professionals EDGE Magazine September 2019

"Never look down on anybody unless you're helping them up" **Jesse Jackson**

Unlocking the Mystery of

Dementia & Dining

Toni Fisk
3 Offers

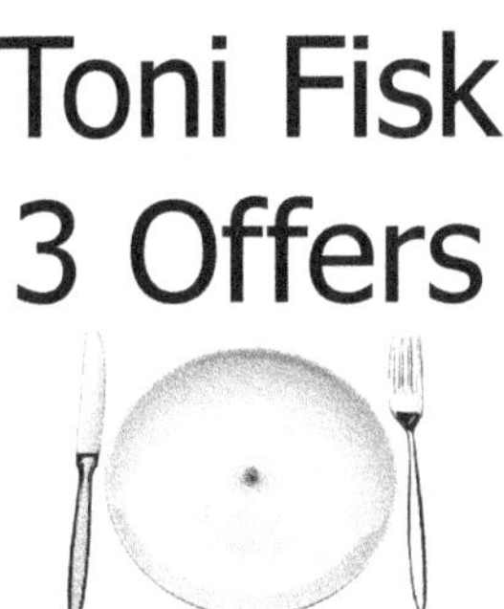

Five Surefire Tips to Boost Communications During Dementia

- Are you confused about dementia and what is happening to your loved one?
- Frustrated with what to do and say when your person living with dementia doesn't "cooperate" with you?
- Do you wish you knew the secret to enjoying life with your loved one despite their dementia?

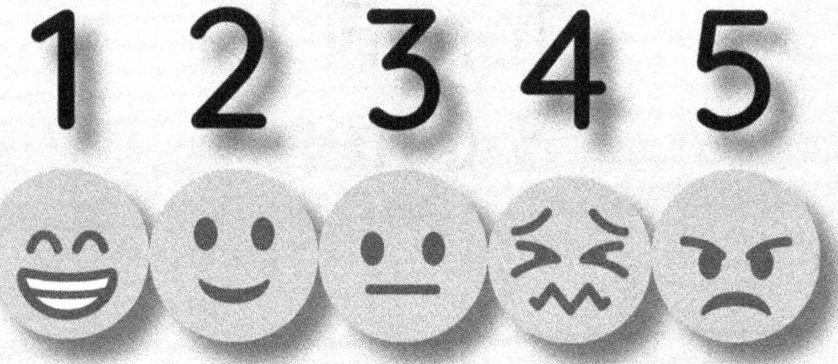

This is a free indispensable handbook for anyone coping with the effects of dementia.

Quickly grasp how you can keep your loved one safe and as happy as humanly possible.

Transform your fear into a joyful existence.

Visit my website's "PUBLICATION" page and click on the FREE button to receive this FREE pdf-get yours now!

https://DinnerWEARhc.info

Professional Dementia Consult

- Do you ever ask yourself, "Am I doing everything I can?"
- Hindsight: "What could I do/have done differently?"
- Wouldn't you like a clear list of things you CAN act upon and change?

After reading this book, do you have other burning questions? Not sure where to turn to for direction and advice? Take advantage of this limited time offer of 30-minute phone consult with Certified Montessori Dementia Care Professional Toni Fisk.

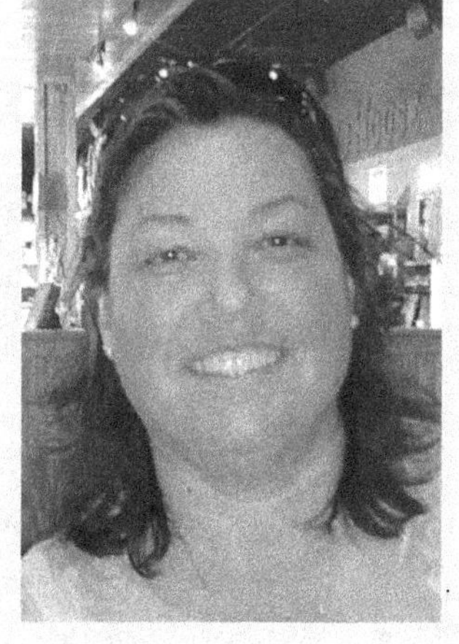

1. Learn to recognize triggers and avoid or deescalate catastrophic behavior.
2. Feel empowered with constructive and compassionate advice.
3. Gain the knowledge to make life simpler and safer for people who have dementia.

Visit my website's "DEMENTIA" page and click on the SCHEDULE AN ASSESSMENT button to book a screening call today!

https://DinnerWEARhc.info

Limited Time Offer—Breakthrough Techniques for Embracing Dementia Workshop

How many times have you said, if I only knew this when/then? Learn from a certified professional the provocative and promising methods detailing what to expect and learn how to handle situations before they become an issue.

- How urgently do you want to improve the quality of YOUR life while not counteracting your loved ones own positive life experience?
- Do you know how to appreciate your person living with dementia's capabilities as well as their losses?
- Why go it alone? Why learn alone when you can use this workshop to improve proper care for your loved one.

Notes

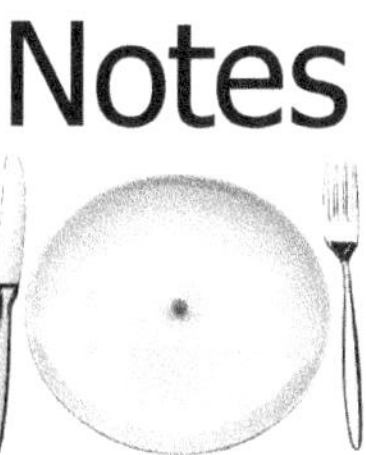

CPSIA information can be obtained
at www.ICGtesting.com
Printed in the USA
BVHW031325290521
608449BV00005B/53